MILITARY SURGICAL MANUALS
NATIONAL RESEARCH COUNCIL

VOLUMES IN THIS SERIES

I. MANUAL OF STANDARD PRACTICE OF PLASTIC AND MAXILLO-
 FACIAL SURGERY

II. OPHTHALMOLOGY AND OTOLARYNGOLOGY

III. ABDOMINAL AND GENITO-URINARY INJURIES

IV. ORTHOPEDIC SUBJECTS

V. BURNS, SHOCK, WOUND HEALING, AND VASCULAR INJURIES

VI. NEUROSURGERY AND THORACIC SURGERY

FOREWORD

THE Medical Department of the Army has been confronted with the necessity for enormous and rapid expansion paralleling that of the armed forces. The state of war has greatly increased the task of furnishing adequate medical care for Army personnel since battle casualties are added to the already wide range of diseases and injuries that must be treated.

Expansion of the medical establishment of the Army is entirely dependent on entry into the service of individuals from civil life. While most reserve officers have had a varying amount of military training, practically all medical officers will encounter problems in the military service entirely foreign to their previous experiences. These problems are by no means confined to those of an administrative nature; many are distinctly professional. The military situation imposes certain restricting factors which render impracticable some procedures that would be considered ideal in civil life. The goal of furnishing the best possible treatment to all individuals is the same in the Army as in civil life, but the means to attain that goal may differ materially.

There has been a marked tendency to specialization within the medical profession since the first World War. This tendency is fundamentally sound but does serve to increase the problems of many individual medical officers in time of war. Specialization cannot be followed to the same degree in the military service as in civil life. While many highly qualified specialists in the various fields of medicine and surgery will serve in like capacities in the Army, this cannot invariably be true. The great burden of medical care will fall on medical officers outside the highly specialized fields. It is thus essential that nearly all medical officers be familiar with the principles of military surgery. Recent advances in therapy have resulted in radical modification of certain principles of treatment that were formerly considered sound.

This series of texts presents in compact form essential up-to-date and reliable information regarding military surgery. The various sections have been written by outstanding authorities in their respective fields. They have been prepared for publication under the auspices of the Division of Medical Sciences of the National Research Council.

These texts will prove a highly valuable source of professional information for any surgeon desiring a knowledge of the principles of military surgery. Their application is not confined to military medicine, for most of the wounds and injuries of modern warfare may be duplicated in civil emergencies. The condensed form and avoidance of debatable points will render them very convenient for quick reference as well as for more mature study.

These volumes represent an important addition to the field of surgical texts. The individuals instrumental in their preparation have made a distinct contribution to civil and military medicine by their assemblage and presentation of this timely professional information.

JAMES C. MAGEE
Major General, U. S. Army
The Surgeon General

The naval medical officer is often faced with medical or surgical situations with which he must deal entirely alone and without the opportunity for consultation and assistance from other members of his profession. He may be the only medical man on a ship in the middle of an ocean, and any surgical emergency must be met by him and him alone. He cannot refer the case to a specialist; he himself must do everything that is necessary. It is important that he have the best assistance that professional books and journals can give him. A volume such as this, which contains practical and essential things, readily accessible, is a real help to a medical officer and patient in this situation.

ROSS T. MCINTIRE
Rear Admiral, Medical Corps
Surgeon General, U. S. Navy

ABDOMINAL AND GENITO-URINARY INJURIES

*Prepared under the Auspices of the Committee on Surgery
of the Division of Medical Sciences of the
National Research Council*

ILLUSTRATED

Philadelphia & London

W. B. SAUNDERS COMPANY

1942

MADE IN U. S. A.

PRESS OF
W. B. SAUNDERS COMPANY
PHILADELPHIA

INTRODUCTION

THIS volume is one of a series developed under the auspices of the Division of Medical Sciences of the National Research Council to furnish the medical departments of the United States Army and Navy with compact presentations of necessary information in the field of military surgery. The individual manuals are prepared under the auspices of the various subcommittees of the Committee on Surgery of the Division of Medical Sciences of the National Research Council and are edited by the Committee on Information.

The first three volumes cover the following subjects: plastic and maxillofacial surgery; ophthalmology and otolaryngology; and abdominal and genito-urinary injuries. Succeeding volumes will contain material on the following: orthopedic subjects (ununited fractures, injuries of the spinal column, compound fractures, and osteomyelitis); burns, shock, wound healing, and vascular injuries; and neurosurgery and thoracic surgery.

The Committee on Surgery includes Drs. Evarts A. Graham, Chairman, Irvin Abell, Donald C. Balfour, George E. Bennett, Warren H. Cole, Frederick A. Coller, Robert H. Ivy, Herman L. Kretschmer, Charles G. Mixter, Howard C. Naffziger, Alton Ochsner, I. S. Ravdin, and Allen O. Whipple. The Committee on Information includes Drs. Morris Fishbein, Chairman, J. J. Bloomfield, John F. Fulton, Richard M. Hewitt, Ira V. Hiscock, Sanford V. Larkey, and Robert N. Nye.

Most of the detail of the editorial work has been done by Dr. Richard M. Hewitt, assisted by Miss M. Katharine Smith, in the Division of Publications, the Mayo Clinic, Rochester, Minnesota.

LEWIS H. WEED, M.D., *Chairman, Division of Medical Sciences of the National Research Council*

MORRIS FISHBEIN, M.D., *Chairman, Committee on Information of the Division of Medical Sciences of the National Research Council*

CHARLES C. HILLMAN, *Brigadier General, U. S. Army; War Department Representative, National Research Council*

CHARLES S. STEPHENSON, *Captain, U. S. Navy Medical Corps; Navy Department Representative, National Research Council*

CONTENTS

ABDOMINAL INJURIES

CHAPTER I
PAGE

ABDOMINAL WOUNDS AND MODERN WARFARE 3

CHAPTER II
GENERAL CONSIDERATIONS 7

CHAPTER III
STUDY AND ESTIMATION OF STATUS OF PATIENTS WITH KNOWN
OR SUSPECTED ABDOMINAL INJURIES 21

CHAPTER IV
GENERAL CARE OF PATIENT, INCLUDING PREOPERATIVE PREP-
ARATION 37

CHAPTER V
SELECTION OF PATIENTS FOR OPERATION 43

CHAPTER VI
PREANESTHETIC PREPARATION AND ANESTHESIA 47

CHAPTER VII
OPERATIVE PROCEDURE 51

CHAPTER VIII
WOUNDS OF SPECIFIC STRUCTURES AND ORGANS 67

CHAPTER IX
POSTOPERATIVE TREATMENT 115

CHAPTER X
COMPLICATIONS 121

CHAPTER XI
RESULTS, MORTALITY, AND STATISTICS 129

CONTENTS

GENITO-URINARY INJURIES

CHAPTER I
PAGE

PRELIMINARY SURVEY OF THE DIAGNOSIS OF WAR INJURIES OF
GENITO-URINARY TRACT IN GENERAL 135

CHAPTER II

INJURIES OF THE KIDNEY AND URETER 149

CHAPTER III

WAR INJURIES OF THE BLADDER 173

CHAPTER IV

CARE OF THE NEUROGENIC BLADDER 187

CHAPTER V

INJURIES OF PENIS AND URETHRA, OF SCROTUM AND CONTENTS,
AND OF PROSTATE GLAND AND SEMINAL VESICLES 203

CHAPTER VI

DO'S AND DON'T'S 217

INDEX 225

ABDOMINAL INJURIES

Prepared by
AMBROSE H. STORCK

*Under the Auspices of
the Committee on Surgery of the Division
of Medical Sciences of the National
Research Council*

EVARTS A. GRAHAM, *Chairman*

IRVIN ABELL

GEORGE E. BENNETT

FREDERICK A. COLLER

HERMAN L. KRETSCHMER

HOWARD C. NAFFZIGER

I. S. RAVDIN

DONALD C. BALFOUR

WARREN H. COLE

ROBERT H. IVY

CHARLES G. MIXTER

ALTON OCHSNER

ALLEN O. WHIPPLE

CONTENTS

CHAPTER I

PAGE

ABDOMINAL WOUNDS AND MODERN WARFARE 3

The Collection, Evacuation, and Disposition of Abdominal
Casualties 3

Surgical Advances, Interchange of Experiences, and Re-
vision of Practice 4

References 4

CHAPTER II

GENERAL CONSIDERATIONS 7

Classification of Abdominal Wounds 7

Incidence of Wounds in Various Parts of Abdomen 7

Projectiles and Other Causes of Penetrating Injuries; Retention of Projectiles 8

Mechanism of Wound Production after Penetration 10

Visceral Injuries without Penetration of Abdominal Wall .. 11

Associated Injuries to Other Parts 13

Shock and Hemorrhage 14

Infection 16

Natural Protective Mechanisms: Spontaneous Recovery
Following Injuries of Hollow and Solid Viscera 17

Controllable Factors Which Influence Mortality, Including
Protection by Armor and Alteration of Intestinal Flora 18

References 19

CHAPTER III

STUDY AND ESTIMATION OF STATUS OF PATIENTS WITH KNOWN
OR SUSPECTED ABDOMINAL INJURIES 21

Symptoms 21

Physical Examination 23

Clinical Laboratory Studies 30

Bacteriologic Studies 32

Roentgenologic Examination 32

Endoscopic Examination 33

Peritoneoscopy 34

Determination of Penetration by Exploration 35

References 35

CHAPTER IV

PAGE

GENERAL CARE OF PATIENT, INCLUDING PREOPERATIVE PREPARATION 37

Treatment of Shock and Hemorrhage 37

Preoperative Antitoxin Therapy 40

References 41

CHAPTER V

SELECTION OF PATIENTS FOR OPERATION 43

Patients Definitely Requiring Operation 43

Patients in Hopeless Condition 43

Patients Not Requiring Operation 44

Borderline Cases 44

CHAPTER VI

PREANESTHETIC PREPARATION AND ANESTHESIA 47

Preanesthetic Preparation 47

Anesthesia 47

References 50

CHAPTER VII

OPERATIVE PROCEDURE 51

Attention to Patient during Operation 51

Types of Incision 52

Order of Operative Procedure 55

Cleansing of Peritoneal Cavity, Peritoneal Lavage, Intraperitoneal Instillation of Bacteriostatic Substances .. 57

Drainage of Peritoneal Cavity 58

Débridement and Épluchage of Wounds 58

Closure of Abdominal Incisions Including Treatment, Drainage, and Dressing of Wound 59

Duration of Operation 64

References 64

CHAPTER VIII

WOUNDS OF SPECIFIC STRUCTURES AND ORGANS 67

Wounds of Peritoneum, Including Wounds Extending into Peritoneal Cavity, without Visceral Injury 67

Wounds of Hollow Alimentary Organs 67

Injuries of Mesentery 87

Injuries to Great Omentum 90

Wounds of Solid Viscera 90

Evisceration Following Abdominal Injury 98

PAGE

Injuries to Major Blood Vessels 99
Wounds of Genito-urinary Organs 100
Abdominothoracic Injuries 107
References 113

CHAPTER IX

POSTOPERATIVE TREATMENT 115
Shock, Hemorrhage, and Hypoproteinemia 115
Dehydration and Demineralization 116
Ileus 117
Wound Infection and Peritonitis 117
Avitaminosis 118
Pulmonary Lesions 118
Thrombosis and Embolism 118
References 118

CHAPTER X

COMPLICATIONS 121
Classification 121
Recognition and Treatment of Residual Abscesses 124
References 128

CHAPTER XI

RESULTS, MORTALITY, AND STATISTICS 129
References 131

ABDOMINAL INJURIES

CHAPTER I

ABDOMINAL WOUNDS AND MODERN WARFARE

ABDOMINAL wounds have always been among the most serious casualties of war. Their successful treatment not only demands judgment and technical skill on the part of the surgeon, but is dependent on thoroughly coordinated medical and military organization.

THE COLLECTION, EVACUATION, AND DISPOSITION OF ABDOMINAL CASUALTIES

The destructiveness and speed of contemporary warfare have greatly increased the problems of collection, evacuation, and treatment of abdominal wounds occurring among armed forces. The care of abdominal wounds aboard ship, while not complicated by problems in collection and transportation, may be difficult because of limited hospital facilities and lack of space. The feasibility of early airplane evacuation of serious casualties to military or civilian hospitals, even at great distance from the area of combat, has been demonstrated in the present war. Transfer by airplane must usually be accomplished in two stages. Small liaison type planes, with a capacity for one or two casualties and capable of landing in a small area, must be used for the initial pick up and transportation to a field to the rear, from which large ambulance transport planes can operate. When airplane transfer of patients with injuries of hollow viscera involves ascent even above 5000 feet, sufficient pressure should be maintained within the cabin to prevent expansion of gas in the stomach and intestine, with resulting extravasation of fluid or gaseous contents of perforated viscera.

Evacuation facilities should, if possible, be so organized that definitive treatment can be accomplished well within the first six hours following injury. When a longer period than this elapses, the chances of recovery are greatly diminished, and if twelve hours elapse, survival is unlikely.

The Mobile Unit

In modern war, in which there is seldom a stabilized line of action, mobile units which can be established in advanced positions are

3

especially necessary. They vary from the small units which provide facilities only for the performance of operations, to the larger ones which include provisions for postoperative care. Transportable units of the latter sort, with a bed capacity as high as 350, have been used in the present war. When an advance is in progress, a method of overcoming the inadequacies of the smaller units is to establish additional units in more advanced positions, while the original ones complete the postoperative care of the patients who cannot be transported to a fixed hospital.

Care of Casualties in Armored Division

Communication between a rapidly advancing armored division and its supporting troops is likely to be impaired or even nonexistent for a period of days, and it may be necessary to provide more than the usual surgical care within the divisional echelon. The mobile hospital may not be able to keep pace with the armored division and, since no unit which cannot be moved within thirty minutes is feasible, operations may necessarily have to be done in trucks. Evacuation of casualties from an advancing armored division to a hospital in the rear can be accomplished by means of quartermaster trucks, which become available from the train. These trucks accommodate sixteen litters racked crosswise.

SURGICAL ADVANCES, INTERCHANGE OF EXPERIENCES, AND REVISION OF PRACTICE

In order that advantage can be taken of experiences gained in the course of a war, accurate studies should be made and records kept concerning all injuries. Notations of what was found and what was done in advanced units should be sent with the patient to the hospitals in the rear. Also, a report on the patient's progress at the latter should be sent to the advanced units.

The so-called radial method of surgical treatment, in which the surgeon is responsible for directing the treatment of the wounded in a given area, both at the advanced stations and in the rear, has some advantages, but in modern warfare usually is not feasible.

REFERENCES

1. Gordon-Taylor, Gordon: The Abdominal Injuries of Warfare. Bristol, John Wright and Sons, Ltd., 1939.
2. Lovelace, W. R., II, and Hargreaves, John: Transportation of Patients by Airplane. J. Aviation Med. 13: 2 (Mar.), 1942.

3. Medical Department of the United States Army in the World War. Washington, D. C., Government Printing Office, 1927, Vol. 11, Part 1.
4. Storck, Ambrose H.: Penetrating Wounds of the Abdomen: an Analysis of Forty-six Personal Cases. Ann. Surg. *111:* 775–819 (May), 1940.
5. Wallace, Cuthbert: War Surgery of the Abdomen. Philadelphia, P. Blakiston's Son and Co., 1918.

CHAPTER II

GENERAL CONSIDERATIONS

CLASSIFICATION OF ABDOMINAL WOUNDS

IN addition to the consideration of wounds as contusions, abrasions, punctured wounds, lacerated wounds, macerated wounds, and so on, abdominal wounds can be classified as follows:

Nonpenetrating Wounds

Wounds of Abdominal Wall.—These include furrowing or gutter wounds, and wounds which perforate part of the abdominal wall and extend tangential to it, without entering the peritoneum; as well as wounds in which the missile lodges in the anterior or lateral abdominal wall, in the retroperitoneal space, or in the muscles of the back.

Subparietal Wounds.—Intraperitoneal injuries without penetration or perforation of the abdominal wall, also referred to as subcutaneous abdominal wounds, include "blast" injuries imparted through air or water, and those due to miscellaneous direct or indirect blunt forces. An increasing proportion of war wounds are of this type.

Penetrating and Perforating Wounds

The differentiation between penetrating and perforating wounds is based on whether or not projectiles have partly or completely traversed the abdomen. However, the terms are often used without respect to strict definition because, in penetrating wounds of the abdominal wall, perforations of viscera may occur and, conversely, perforating wounds of the abdominal wall may be accompanied only by simple penetration of the surface of a solid viscus, or of one wall of a hollow viscus.

INCIDENCE OF WOUNDS IN VARIOUS PARTS OF ABDOMEN

The comparative rarity in hospital of patients with wounds in the median line is due to the presence there of the great vessels, injury to which usually causes immediate death. The collection of wounds

7

toward the sides of the body in the war of 1914–1918 was due partly to the fact that men in trenches were more or less protected from the front and the rear, whereas the sides of their bodies were open to enfilade fire.

PROJECTILES AND OTHER CAUSES OF PENETRATING INJURIES; RETENTION OF PROJECTILES

Projectiles as Causes of Abdominal Wounds

Bullets.—Bullets are relatively less frequently the cause of injury than formerly, but wounds caused by fire from machine guns

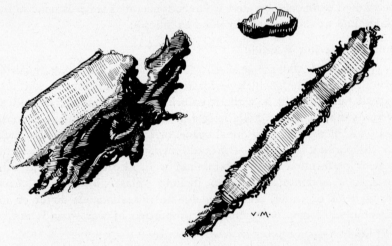

Fig. 1.—Fragments of high-explosive shells used in the present war. Fragments of this sort, along with bullets, are responsible for most of the wounds in contemporary warfare. Because of their irregular shape, fragments of high-explosive shells cause ragged lacerations, and the larger ones are likely to be retained if traveling at low velocity.

and by automatic rifles and pistols are still numerous. Whether from inherent instability, or from hitting an object, bullets frequently spin, and in some cases a relatively large entrance wound is produced.

Shell Fragments.—Shell fragments are of all shapes and sizes, and cause injury either by penetration or, in the instance of large, low velocity fragments, by blunt force. The fragments which produce wounds requiring surgical treatment generally do not exceed 1½ inches (3.8 cm.) in greatest diameter.

High-Explosive Shells.—These shells have largely replaced shrapnel. The velocity of the fragments depends both on the "remaining velocity" and on the disruptive charge, and the fragments fly out principally in an obliquely forward or lateral direction. The form of the fragments depends on the type of shell: if the shell is segmented, the pieces are more or less quadrilateral; if the shell is not segmented, the fragments are still more or less quadrilateral and have extremely sharp and ragged edges. It is estimated that a very effective man-killing weight of splinters from high-explosive shells is about 25 gm., although splinters even lighter than 10 gm. may be lethal if they strike near the point of explosion (Fig. 1).

Shrapnel.—Now rarely used, these shells are usually exploded in the air by means of a time fuse. Shrapnel shells and the balls with which they are filled vary in size. The penetrating power of the balls is influenced by the velocity of the shell at the time of explosion. Some shells are of a combined high-explosive and shrapnel type.

Shell Caps.—Shell caps of various types sometimes cause contusions without perforation and are among the largest fragments responsible for abdominal injuries.

Grenades and Bombs.—Although bombs have often been extemporized from metal boxes filled with an explosive, scrap iron, cobblers' nails, screws, and so forth, they are usually made of iron, the surface of which is grooved, so that on explosion they break up into quadrilateral fragments. Some bomb fragments, however, are no larger than a matchhead but have great penetrating power in the immediate vicinity of the explosion.

Trench-Mortar Bombs.—Of various shapes, this type of projectile consists essentially of a very large high-explosive charge within a comparatively thin containing envelope, which often bursts into ragged, large, as well as minute, fragments.

Aerial Bombs.—Modern aerial bombs are of several types and are generally classifiable as fragmentation, demolition, armor-piercing, incendiary and gas bombs, as well as aerial mine bombs. They vary greatly in size, and the injuries caused by them frequently are not due to the fragments from the bombs but to secondary projectiles which their explosions displace. Burns produced by incendiary bombs, and the lesions caused by gas bombs, complicate the management of the injuries due to mechanical trauma.

Retention of Projectiles

Bullets.—Causes for the retention of bullets are not always determinable, as bullets fired even at short range sometimes remain within the body. Ricochet or passage through an object before the bullet reaches the abdominal wall often accounts for their retention.

Shells.—Due to their frequent large size and irregular shape, fragments from high-explosive shells cause a large proportion of abdominal wounds, and many of the fragments are retained.

Bombs and Grenades.—Fragments from bombs and grenades are often retained because of their relatively low velocity.

Miscellaneous Objects.—Splinters of wood, fragments of structural steel, or pieces of brick, glass and mortar, are among objects likely to be retained.

Wandering Missiles.—Wandering of missiles is rare. However, "healed-in" metal splinters are frequently not embedded in firm connective tissue but are surrounded by loose granulation tissue, thus not only accounting for the accumulation of fluid around them, but also explaining the fact that the projectile may be displaced from its original position to a new location where aseptic inflammation may again be set up.

Additional Causes of Penetrating Abdominal Injury

Penetrating wounds of the abdomen also may be produced by bayonets, pikes, knives, and so on. Bayonet wounds seldom are observed in a hospital, for they usually prove immediately fatal.

MECHANISM OF WOUND PRODUCTION AFTER PENETRATION

Wounds of various types, sustained by the same patient, have been accounted for by "spinning," "tumbling," or rotation of the projectile, or have been ascribed to a bursting effect, when it has seemed impossible that a missile pursuing a straight course could cause such multiform injuries. In the instance of bullets, support of the rotation theory is furnished by the fact that many bullets causing such injuries are retained, implying that their flight is unstable at the moment of penetration. Convincing evidence concerning the bursting effect, or "paper-bag" theory, is lacking. The different types of wounds are also due to the varied disposition of the small intestine. Under normal circumstances some segments of the small intestine are distended with air, while others are collapsed, and if a bullet strikes a dilated portion it will cause a perforation, whereas if it strikes a collapsed portion the diameter of the bullet is great enough to divide the bowel entirely. This concept is supported by observations on injuries of the large bowel, where perforations are much more common than are extensive tears or complete division. When total division of the large intestine does occur, it is in the transverse, descending, or pelvic colon, which is often collapsed. The intestine, especially the small bowel, may be torn away from its mesentery over a distance of several feet, without perforation. The explosive effect of some injuries of the distended urinary bladder is a simple hydrodynamic one, being due to the force exerted on incompressible fluid in a confined space. The absence of such effects in the instance of injuries to blood vessels is probably due to the indefinite continuity of fluid above and below the stricken spot, and to the strength and elasticity of both arteries and veins.

VISCERAL INJURIES WITHOUT PENETRATION OF ABDOMINAL WALL

Injuries to abdominal viscera, without penetration of the abdominal wall, are fairly frequent and are designated as *subparietal* or *subcutaneous* wounds. The normal turgor of the *solid intra-abdominal viscera* makes these relatively inelastic organs more liable to injuries by blunt force. *Hollow viscera,* such as the intestine and the urinary bladder or gallbladder, are more liable to injury by blunt force if distended by gas or fluid. Contributing factors in injuries caused by indirect violence are limitation of mobility by a mesentery, by blood vessels, or by retroperitoneal fixation.

Although the adoption of motorized equipment has reduced the number of subparietal injuries due to kicks by mules and horses, many casualties now result from being hit or rolled over by, or thrown about in, machines. Injuries to hollow or solid viscera resulting from compression between the steering wheel or other parts of motorized equipment, and the patient's spinal column, are likely to be incurred by drivers of mechanized equipment. Rupture of viscera without penetration of the abdominal wall may be caused by a blow on the abdomen with the butt of a rifle; by falls; by large shell fragments; by flying pieces of wood or other objects; or through crushing by timbers, brick, mortar, structural steel, or earth (Fig. 2).

Abdominal viscera may be damaged by inbent overlying ribs, or by indriven spicules of bone. Wounds of this sort to the liver, the spleen, and the kidneys are frequently caused by fractured ribs. In pelvic fractures the small intestine and, less commonly, the cecum, the descending and the ascending colon, the pelvic colon, the rectum, and the urinary bladder may be injured by bone fragments. Even though a projectile has not penetrated the peritoneal membrane, it is important to consider the possibility of perforation by bone, as the small holes caused by bone splinters are frequently not noticed even when the abdomen is explored.

"Blast" injuries, although more frequently involving the lungs and tympanic membranes, may also cause subparietal damage to abdominal viscera, including the liver and the intestine. These injuries are usually due to the rapid and extreme changes in air pressure which follow explosion of large bombs, particularly aerial bombs or high explosive shells. There are experimental evidences that in air blast injuries it is the pressure wave which causes impact on the body wall and that this effect can be prevented or diminished if the body is padded or shielded with a material which can take up and disperse

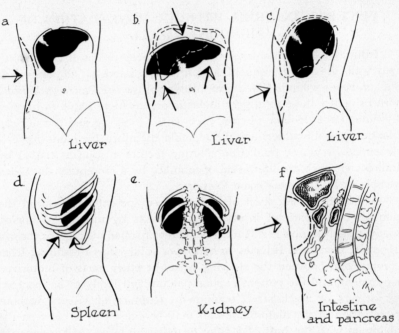

Fig. 2.—Diagrams illustrating the mechanism of subparietal injuries to abdominal viscera, caused by the forces indicated by arrows. The size, location, and friability of the liver and, to a lesser extent, of the spleen and kidneys make them susceptible to injury by blunt force. Fixation by a mesentery or by a vascular pedicle are also important elements in the mechanism of such injuries to both solid and hollow viscera. Compression may be exerted by intact ribs, or underlying viscera may be penetrated by fractured ribs. Air and water "blast" wave compression injuries have assumed increased importance in modern warfare.

the pressure wave. In the instance of men partially submerged in water, compression abdominal injuries may be caused by the blast wave set up in the surrounding fluid by a depth charge, torpedo, or the underwater explosion of a shell.

Subparietal injuries of hollow viscera include contusions of the wall, minute perforations, extensive lacerations, or even complete division of the bowel or its mesentery. Solid visceral lesions of this sort comprise subcapsular rupture, slight tears, and extensive lacerations; such injuries are often associated with a subcapsular hematoma. The organs most often ruptured are the liver, spleen, kidneys, pancreas, and small intestine. The mesentery may be torn away from a segment of bowel. The fixation of the duodenum makes it likely to be ruptured by crushing wounds of the abdomen.

Subparietal ruptures of solid or hollow viscera are frequently overlooked, and the prognosis in cases of such injury is generally poor, for it is often not until shock and hemorrhage, or even peritonitis, have become established, that the possibility of intra-abdominal trauma is suspected.

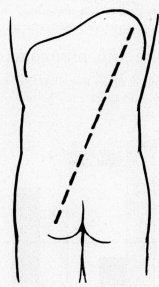

Fig. 3.—Diagram indicating the transabdominal course of a missile after entering at a point remote from the abdominal wall. Abdominal viscera are frequently injured by missiles which enter through the buttocks, perineum, thigh, or thorax.

Other groups of cases in which abdominal visceral injury may occur without perforation of the parietes are those in which missiles enter either via the thorax, or after first traversing the buttocks, sacrum, perineum, or thighs (Fig. 3).

ASSOCIATED INJURIES TO OTHER PARTS

The steel helmet has reduced the incidence of associated injuries of the *head and neck*. Armor for the protection of the chest and abdomen would, if found practicable, reduce the number of complicating injuries of the *chest* and *spinal column*. Armor for at least partial protection of the *extremities* also has been suggested.

Burns produced by chemicals, including vesicant and other gases, or by heat and flames from shells, incendiary bombs, or flame throwers, not only increase the degree of shock but complicate or delay attention to abdominal injuries.

When multiple wounds exist, the abdominal wound usually should be treated before other injuries but, under some circumstances, the complicating conditions, such as the effects of *gas*, may require first attention. Simultaneous care of injuries in various parts of the body by multiple surgical teams should sometimes be given, while in other cases, the nature and extent of the *associated injuries* preclude anything but completely conservative management.

SHOCK AND HEMORRHAGE

The degree of shock is often not directly proportional to the extent of anatomic injury, and there may be one or more of the several

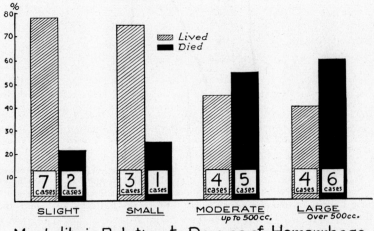

Mortality in Relation to Degree of Hemorrhage

Fig. 4.—Graphic representation of the direct relationship between the amount of hemorrhage and the mortality in a series of forty-six cases of penetrating bullet and stab wounds of the abdomen. Comparison with Fig. 5, which shows the average number of perforations in relationship to mortality, emphasizes the greater importance of hemorrhage in determining the outcome in penetrating abdominal wounds.

following reasons for this discrepancy: The patient's general condition at the time of injury, as influenced by loss of sleep; nervous, mental, or physical strain; exposure to cold and wet; thirst, hunger, or general fatigue, all of which may have increased his susceptibility to shock. The wound may have involved an organ or region in which injury is followed by severe shock. Spillage into the peritoneal cavity of even small amounts of blood is usually followed by a greater degree of shock than would follow the external loss of an equal amount of blood. Shock may occur soon after receipt of the wound or may develop gradually. It may pass off shortly, may persist and even deepen, or may reappear after a period of improvement.

The absence of a direct ratio between the number of perforations of solid or hollow viscera and the death rate, compared with the constant, direct relationship between the amount of hemorrhage and the mortality, is indicated in Figs. 4 and 5. Massive hemorrhage in association with abdominal wounds may be due to: (1) *Perforation of vessels in the abdominal wall,* most commonly one of the deep epigas-

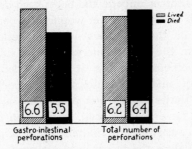

Fig. 5.—Graphic representation of the average number of visceral perforations in relationship to the mortality in a series of forty-six penetrating bullet and stab wounds of the abdomen. Comparison with Fig. 4 reveals that the mortality is more directly related to the degree of hemorrhage than to the number of perforations.

tric arteries. The combined intraperitoneal, subperitoneal, and external bleeding from an injury of one of these arteries may prove fatal. (2) *Bleeding from the great vessels of the abdomen.* Although such injuries usually cause death before the patient reaches the hospital, continued or recurrent bleeding from the vena cava, the iliac, renal, or splenic veins, or large branches of the superior mesenteric artery may be found at the time of operation. (3) *Hemorrhage arising from solid organs,* such as the liver, spleen, and kidneys. These organs bleed freely and when the injury occurs near large vessels in the hilar regions, fatal hemorrhage is frequent. (4) *Injury of the omentum.* Bleeding from omental vessels is often responsible for most of the blood in the peritoneal cavity at the time of operation. (5) *Wounds of large mesenteric blood vessels.* The bleeding may occur directly into the peritoneal cavity, or injury to these vessels may be followed by the formation of hematomas in the retroperitoneal spaces or between the leaves of the mesentery.

Bleeding between the leaves of the mesentery, or *into extraperitoneal spaces,* is sometimes practically impossible to control, because the bleeding point is obscured by the resulting hematoma. Large amounts of blood may be extravasated into the retroperitoneal space, and is frequently followed by intestinal ileus.

Bleeding from the wall proper of the *stomach or intestine,* is not usually great in amount, but considerable bleeding may occur from injury to the vessels on the surface of the stomach or the large bowel.

INFECTION

Bacterial contamination, either from spillage of gastro-intestinal contents, or from sources outside the body such as soil or dirty clothing, may involve either the original wound, the peritoneum, the retroperitoneal tissue or the operative wound. Residual abscesses frequently develop in the subphrenic space, the subhepatic space, the iliac fossae, the rectovesical space, or between loops of intestine.

The degree of infection which follows perforation of gastrointestinal viscera varies even when practically identical segments of stomach or bowel have been injured. In addition to the factor of host resistance, this inconsistency is related to the amount and character of food ingested before the injury was incurred, as well as to variations in the intestinal bacterial flora of different individuals.

Gastric wounds, if small, and especially if located near the lesser curvature, or at the cardiac end of the stomach, are followed by little spilling, whereas if the wound is large and near the greater curvature, the entire contents of the stomach may be emptied into the peritoneal cavity. Extravasation of the gastric contents shortly following eating or drinking may be more or less harmful, depending on the character of what was ingested. Milk and uncooked food, or food contaminated by soiled hands, is particularly dangerous, and poor oral hygiene and low gastric acidity also unfavorably influence the effects produced by spilling of gastric contents.

Some parts of the small intestine are usually empty, otherwise spilling of considerable amounts of material from this portion of the alimentary tract would be even more common and would more frequently lead to severe peritonitis. Effusion of the contents of the duodenum or jejunum is not usually serious, unless perforation occurs while these viscera are filled. The character and abundance of the bacterial flora of the ileum make perforations of this part of the intestine particularly dangerous, and were it not for the occasionally firm consistency of the contents of the ileum, and the usual deposition of its spilled contents in the lower part of the abdomen, such perforations would be even more highly fatal.

Because of the normally solid or semisolid consistency of the contents of the colon, diffuse peritoneal contamination is less likely to occur after its penetration than when the small intestine is perforated, especially if the wound is small. An additional factor, which influences the outcome following injuries of the large intestine, is that a great number of the bacteria in it are dead.

NATURAL PROTECTIVE MECHANISMS: SPONTANEOUS RECOVERY FOLLOWING INJURIES OF HOLLOW AND SOLID VISCERA

The probability of spontaneous recovery following penetrating wounds, especially of hollow viscera, is *too remote to warrant elective dependence on nonoperative management.* There are, however, several natural protective mechanisms which usually develop when either hollow or solid viscera have been injured. A fall in blood pressures, due to shock and loss of blood, and the normal coagulating mechanism, tend to arrest hemorrhage. Eversion and edema of the mucosa following intestinal injuries often effectively plug the smaller wounds. Sealing of penetrations in hollow viscera may be effected by blood clots, omentum, contiguous loops of bowel, nearby solid viscera, the abdominal wall, or later by fibrin. Spontaneous arrest of hemorrhage and limitation of spillage from the gastro-intestinal tract often maintain patients in reasonably good condition for many hours. Were it not for such protective mechanisms, the mortality in cases of abdominal injury would be much higher. However, even when augmented by the best nonoperative methods of treatment, these processes cannot be depended on in cases in which there are gaping wounds in the intestine, and they are often incapable of entirely arresting primary hemorrhage, or of averting secondary hemorrhage. After twelve or more hours have elapsed since injury, operation, with its attendant shock and breaking down of protective barriers, is almost invariably followed by an early fatal outcome. Under such circumstances the possibility of recovery, remote as it is, is greater if the natural protective mechanisms are relied on without operative intervention.

Recovery following spontaneous development of a fecal fistula, when a perforation of the intestine has not been surgically repaired, is an additional example of a spontaneous mechanism which some-times protects patients who reach the hospital late, or who for other reasons are not operated on.

CONTROLLABLE FACTORS WHICH INFLUENCE MOR-TALITY, INCLUDING PROTECTION BY ARMOR AND ALTERATION OF INTESTINAL FLORA

Abdominal wounds are so highly fatal that it is important to con-sider methods by which their incidence may be reduced, or their destructive character lessened.

Armor

The value of body armor as a means of protection, especially against shell and bomb fragments which are traveling at low velocity, and against small caliber bullets, is suggested by the many instances in which penetration of missiles has been prevented by thick cloth-ing, belt buckles, or a note book or metal mirror in a soldier's pocket. Furthermore, at least partial protection against blast injuries is afforded by clothing the body in a material which can disperse the pressure wave.

Requirements for armor are that it be not too heavy or cumber-some, or otherwise unacceptable to the wearer. Although effective armor which partially meets these requirements has been developed and used to a limited extent in modern warfare, employment of this form of protection will probably be restricted to special troops. In desert warfare armor becomes extremely hot, and the overheating and excessive sweating which it causes adds to fatigue due to support-ing the extra weight. An additional objection to body armor is that it affords protection to vermin. The contention that the wearing of armor induces an "oyster complex" hardly seems justified. Although motorized equipment has increased the feasibility of body armor being worn by troops on the move, the increased use of tanks and armored vehicles has in a measure reduced the possible need for individual body armor.

Some of the substances which have been suggested or studied in respect to their adaptability as armor are: chain mail; wire mesh or net; sheet metal, notably manganese steel, chromium steel, silicon nickel steel; aluminum alloys; rubber; laminated metal and rubber; woven silk; cork; compressed canvas; leather; asbestos; paper; cotton; rayon; bakelite and other plastics; miscellaneous fibers, hemp, sisal, hair, flax, kapok; and the gum, balata.

Emptying of Bowel and Bladder

Since the mortality of penetrating wounds of the abdomen is related to the amount and character of gastro-intestinal spillage, it is desirable that the alimentary tract at the time of penetration be as nearly empty as possible. Troops about to go into action should refrain from eating immediately beforehand and should, when possible, evacuate the lower bowel shortly before combat. It is also advisable that the urinary bladder be emptied, because if it is distended it is not only more likely to be injured but the wound is often of a bursting character.

Alteration of Intestinal Flora

The fact that the administration of cultures of lactobacilli in the form of acidophilus milk can almost entirely eliminate pathogenic organisms from the intestine within a few days, suggests the value of transforming the intestinal flora of troops about to go into action, so that severe peritonitis would be less likely to follow perforation of the bowel. The possibility of greatly reducing the number of living micro-organisms in the alimentary tract by means of the oral administration of sulfonamide drugs has been demonstrated and, were it not for their toxic effects, the use of these drugs might contribute to the prevention of peritonitis.

REFERENCES

1. Breden, N. P., d'Abreu, A. L., and King, D. P.: Sudden Compression Injuries of the Adomen at Sea. Brit. M. J. *1:* 144–146 (Jan. 31), 1942.
2. Gage, I. M.: Personal communication to the author.
3. Harkins, H. N.: Treatment of Shock in Wartime. War Med. *1:* 520–535 (July), 1941.
4. Kekwick, A., Marriott, H. L., Maycock, W. d'A., and Whitby, L. E. H.: Diagnosis and Treatment of Secondary Shock; a Study of 24 Cases. Lancet. *1:* 99–103 (Jan.), 1941.
5. Lohmüller, W., Jr.: Der Steckschuss (zugl. ein Beitrag zur Frage der Teschosswanderung). München. med. Wchnschr. *87:* 829–832 (Aug.), 1940.
6. Marshall, E. K., Jr., Bratton, A. C., White, H. J., and Litchfield, J. T., Jr.: Sulfanilylguanidine; Chemotherapeutic Agent for Intestinal Infections. Bull. Johns Hopkins Hosp. *67:* 163–188 (Sept.), 1940.
7. Odelberg, Axel: Surgical War Experiences. Brit. M. J. *2:* 43–46 (July), 1940.
8. Rettger, L. F., and Cheplin, H. A.: A Treatise on the Transformation of the Intestinal Flora with Special Reference to the Implantation of Bacillus Acidophilus. New Haven, Yale University Press, 1921.
9. Storck, Ambrose H.: Abdominal Injuries; Preventive and Prophylactic Aspects. Ann. Surg. *113:* 720–729 (May), 1941.
10. The Medical Department of the United States Army in the World War: Cited before.

11. Wallace, Cuthbert: Cited before.
12. Walter, K. M.: The Protection of the Soldier in Warfare. Proc. Roy. Soc.
        Med. *33:* 607, 1940.
13. Zuckerman, S.: Experimental Study of Blast Injuries to the Lungs. Lancet.
        2: 219–224 (Aug.), 1940.

STUDY AND ESTIMATION OF STATUS OF PATIENTS WITH KNOWN OR SUSPECTED ABDOMINAL INJURIES

APPRAISAL of patients with abdominal injury includes estimation not only of *abdominal damage,* but also of the degree of *shock, hemorrhage,* and *peritoneal contamination,* and of the character of *associated injuries.* It is desirable to know the circumstances under which the injury occurred, the cause of the injury, the *period of time elapsed,* and the treatment already given.

The *least number of clinical and laboratory studies* which permit determination of the patient's condition are to be employed. The location and character of the injury, or evidence of internal hemorrhage, may make it obvious that visceral injury exists. When there is doubt concerning the occurrence of penetration, or when clinical signs of shock or hemorrhage are lacking, roentgenologic examination and laboratory studies may be necessary.

SYMPTOMS

Pain

The degree and character of pain following wounds of the abdomen *vary greatly.* Neither the presence or absence, nor the amount, of pain necessarily indicates the existence or the extent of abdominal injury. Some pain is ordinarily present and, although usually felt immediately after injury, in the midst of battle it is sometimes unnoticed until considerable time has elapsed. This is probably due not alone to excitement, but also to the fact that pain in abdominal injuries does not depend so much on visceral trauma as on the amount of hemorrhage or spillage of hollow visceral contents. Extravasation of acid gastric juice may immediately cause excruciating pain, whereas perforation of the cecum, with spilling of only a small amount of solid or semisolid material, may cause practically no discomfort, especially if there is little or no associated hemorrhage. The amount of pain following injuries which involve only the abdominal wall is frequently greater than when the peritoneum has been penetrated. A localized painful region distant from the point of entrance may indicate the region in which the missile is lodged. The frequent painlessness of abdominal injuries accounts for the fact that soldiers with extensive wounds, and even with evisceration of abdominal organs, have continued in action or have walked considerable distances after being wounded. Trauma to the lumbar plexus sometimes causes pain in the corresponding lower extremity, so that the wound may be thought to involve the thigh or leg rather than the abdomen.

When large objects, such as shell fragments or shell caps, bluntly injure the abdomen, a sensation is experienced similar to that produced by any violent blow. Small projectiles sometimes cause a sensation as if a blow had been sustained by a large object but the sensation produced by them is usually sharp or stabbing.

Pain may be either transient or persistent and may be accompanied by collapse. When intestinal evisceration has occurred, there may be cramping peristaltic pain, but adynamic ileus usually rapidly involves not only the extruded loop but also the bowel retained within the abdomen. Intraperitoneal hemorrhage or the escape of gas into the subdiaphragmatic regions may cause pain referred to the root of the neck. Normally there is not sufficient gas in either the small or the large intestine to produce this latter symptom.

Testicular pain has been a frequent symptom of patients who have sustained compression injuries of the abdomen while in water near the site of explosion of a depth charge.

Injuries in other parts of the body sometimes so completely direct the patient's attention to these parts that he ignores the pain due to the abdominal injury. Whether the patient has or has not received morphine must be taken into consideration in assaying pain.

Nausea and Vomiting

The presence or absence of nausea and vomiting *cannot be depended on* to indicate whether intraperitoneal injury has occurred. The amount of vomiting is influenced by the injured person's normal tendency to become nauseated and to vomit. Although severe nausea and vomiting may accompany injury to practically any abdominal region or viscus, particularly the stomach, esophagus, and kidneys, these symptoms may be absent, regardless of the location or character of the wound, the amount of spillage of contents of the alimentary tract, or the extent of either intraperitoneal or extraperitoneal hemorrhage. Hematemesis often does not accompany injuries to the stomach.

Miscellaneous Symptoms

Air hunger usually follows considerable loss of blood and, when there has been extensive hemorrhage, it may be evident to the examiner.

Dyspnea, although most often observed in cases of abdomino-thoracic injuries, may be pronounced even when no thoracic injury accompanies the abdominal wound.

Vesical or rectal tenesmus sometimes follows injury to the urinary bladder or to the rectum. One or more bowel movements may occur shortly after an abdominal injury, even though there has been no wound of the rectum or anus. Although the material excreted by bowel may contain blood or be streaked or coated with blood, early and complete spontaneous hemostasis often prevents the appearance of gross blood. Passage of blood by rectum and the vomiting of blood have been frequent signs of water blast wave injuries of the abdomen.

PHYSICAL EXAMINATION

Physical examination, even though quickly performed, must be sufficiently complete to reveal associated injuries and to detect wounds produced by missiles which may have entered the abdomen via remote regions, such as the buttocks, thighs, perineum or thorax.

Inspection

General Appearance.—Patients with abdominal wounds usually seem ill in proportion to the extent of the injury, but their appearance is influenced by the time elapsed since injury, by variations in individual reaction to an equal degree of pain, by the amount of shock and hemorrhage, and by first aid attention, such as the administration of morphine. The patient may be extremely restless and excited but oftener is quiet, drowsy, or even apathetic, because of loss of sleep or sustained physical and mental exhaustion. In many instances, the patient's desire to secure rest and to sleep supersedes any concern about his wounds. The color may be good, or there may be pallor and occasionally even cyanosis, especially if there is thoracic injury. Perspiration is frequently profuse. Dyspnea and rapid respiration are usually present when there is a thoracic lesion. Air hunger may be detectable by inspection. A calm facial expression, perfect composure and interest in the surroundings may reflect a phlegmatic disposition, and such an appearance *can be misleading,* for it is often manifested by those most seriously injured.

Inspection of the abdomen usually reveals diminution or absence of the normal movement timed with respiration. Breathing which is wholly or principally thoracic in type is sometimes observed when the injury is limited to the abdominal wall, but absence of abdominal excursion suggests intraperitoneal extension of the wound. A bluish area rarely may be seen in the region of the umbilicus when there is a large amount of blood in the peritoneal cavity.

In association with various types of blast injury, as well as in many cases of nonpenetrating injury of the abdomen due to blunt or indirect force, there are no surface evidences of injury. This may also be true when a penetrating missile enters at a point remote from the abdomen and is retained. Inspection of the abdominal wall, however, usually furnishes information concerning wounds of entrance or exit, and may reveal discharge of urine or feces, or external bleeding. A plug of omentum in, or protruding through, a wound at once indicates that the peritoneum has been perforated. A knuckle or loop of either intact or injured intestine, or a portion of the stomach, spleen or liver, sometimes will be found projecting into or completely through the wound in the abdominal wall. Occasionally a bullet or shell fragment can be seen in an open wound, and projectiles lying beneath the skin can be detected by the bulging which they cause, especially when surrounded by a hematoma. Subcutaneous rupture of a muscle of the abdominal wall may be indicated by a hematoma at the site of injury.

Prominence of the flanks occasionally may be caused by intraperitoneal extravasation of blood and intestinal contents. Distention of the abdomen and a corrugated appearance of the abdominal wall, produced by dilated loops of bowel, are signs which are observed only late, after peritonitis and ileus have appeared. When the spinal cord has been injured, the distended urinary bladder may cause prominence of the lower part of the abdomen.

Determination of Course of Projectiles, Based on Study of External Wounds, Including Consideration of Effect of Posture.—Study of points of entrance and exit, or even of a wound of entrance alone, can be helpful in determining whether or not peritoneal penetration has occurred, especially in the instance of bullet wounds. The wound of entrance is ordinarily smaller than the caliber of the bullet, whereas the point of exit is usually more irregular and larger than the wound of entrance. A concentric area of abrasion and contusion surrounding the point of entrance indicates that the bullet has taken a straight course, and that the underlying viscera in the region have probably been injured; if the abraded area is to the right of the wound, it signifies that the missile has passed from right to left. Obliquely directed bullets undermine the skin opposite the area of surface

abrasion and, since this is increased with the obliquity, the more superficial the bullet track, the larger the superficial contusion and the
greater the undermining. This is of importance in estimating the
extent and direction of superficial, nonpenetrating wounds of the abdomen which cause pain and at times nausea, vomiting, tenderness and
rigidity. Wounds produced by irregular or jagged projectiles yield
much less definite or dependable information than that which can be
gained in the instance of wounds caused by bullets (Fig. 6).

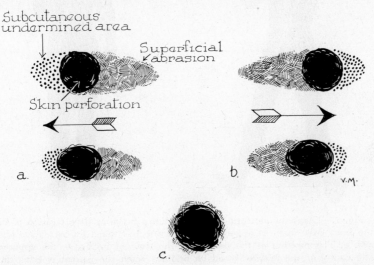

Fig. 6.—Drawing illustrating various types of external wounds in relation
to the courses taken by bullets. If the area of abrasion is to the right of the
edge of the wound, it signifies that the missile has passed from right to left, *a*,
and vice versa, *b*, if the area of abrasion is to the left of the edge of the wound.
A concentric area of cutaneous abrasion indicates that the bullet has taken a
straight course, *c*. Furthermore, the amount of undermining beneath the edge of
the wound opposite the area of abrasion may also indicate the obliquity of the
course of the missile.

The apparently bizarre courses of projectiles, often erroneously
ascribed to deflection or ricochet, may be due to a bent over, crouched,
or partially turned position at the time of injury. Also, the shift of
position of organs from that which existed at the time of injury to
that which exists when the patient is lying on the operating table,
may be considerable. The changed position of viscera during various
phases of respiration also sometimes accounts for seemingly erratic
courses of missiles (Figs. 7, 8).

The intraperitoneal entrance of a projectile through the *buttocks,
thighs, sacral region,* or *perineum* is often overlooked. Wounds of this

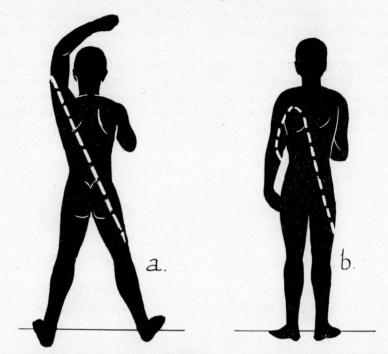

Fig. 7.—Diagrams indicating that variations in the relative position of parts of the body may make it appear that a missile has taken an extremely erratic course. *a,* The position of the patient at the time of injury; *b,* the apparently erratic course of the missile, based on findings when the patient is lying on an operating table.

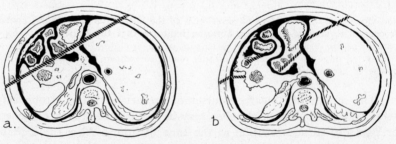

Fig. 8.—Diagrammatic representation of the shift in the relative position of abdominal viscera and wound tracks caused by a change of posture or by respiration. *a,* Relative position of viscera when wound was inflicted; *b,* when examined during operation.

sort are frequently associated with injuries of the pelvic blood vessels, the rectum, the pelvic colon, and sometimes loops of small bowel. More rarely the bladder, the ureters, the posterior urethra, and the prostate gland may be injured. Even very small shell splinters or other missiles may cause extensive lacerated wounds of viscera or tears of large blood vessels.

Muerte Subperitoneal.—In the condition termed "muerte subperitoneal" (subperitoneal death), there are premonitory symptoms of coldness of the extremities, cold sweat, cyanosis and feeble and rapid pulse but they are not accompanied by signs of peritonitis. A particularly grave sign is semierection of the penis, which is reported to be always followed by death. The cause of this symptom is probably hemorrhage into the retroperitoneal spaces around the root of the mesentery.

Palpation

Palpation of Skin.—Except when there is elevation of temperature due to peritonitis or wound infection, the skin is usually moist and cool. Subnormal surface temperature is frequently associated with subnormal oral and rectal temperatures.

Pulse.—The *rate and quality* of the pulse are ordinarily related to the degree of shock and hemorrhage. The pulse is frequently rapid and thready but a slow pulse does not necessarily indicate the absence of serious abdominal injury. Bradycardia accompanying injuries of the liver and biliary tract has been ascribed to the absorption of bile extravasated into the peritoneal cavity. Visceral perforation, particularly when involving hollow viscera, and if unassociated with hemorrhage, shock or infection, may not cause increase in rate or impairment of quality of the pulse. The prognosis in cases in which the pulse rate does not exceed *100 beats per minute* is generally good, whereas death frequently occurs when the pulse rate is 120 or higher. A rapid pulse rate at the time the patient is first seen may be partly due to pain or excitement. Slowing of the pulse often follows even a short period of rest and quiet. It has been stated that a rapid pulse, a pulse that does not fall, or a rising pulse, is an indication for operation, but *changes* in the pulse are frequently undependable, and relatively late in indicating the existence, as well as the progress, of shock and hemorrhage.

Tenderness.—Evaluation of abdominal tenderness is difficult. Tenderness due to a wound of the abdominal wall is ordinarily *localized*, whereas tenderness due to visceral injury and extravasation of blood, or fluid gastro-intestinal contents is usually diffuse. If only a small amount of blood or gastro-intestinal contents spills into the peritoneal cavity, there may be little or no tenderness. A tender tract sometimes can be traced, corresponding to the course of a missile in the abdominal wall, and an area of circumscribed tenderness may indicate the resting point of a missile, either in the abdominal wall or in the abdomen. Tenderness is sometimes due to distention of the urinary bladder.

Rigidity.—The degree and location of rigidity can lead to *false judgment* in respect to abdominal injury.

Abdominal rigidity not only follows penetration of the abdomen, but frequently accompanies *low thoracic injuries,* and is usually associated with wounds of the *abdominal wall,* the *pelvic floor,* and even of the *thigh.* The amount of blood, as well as the character and volume of gastro-intestinal spillage, determines the degree and extent of rigidity. Spilling of solid intestinal contents is usually followed by slight or undetectable rigidity while the presence in the peritoneal cavity of even a small amount of irritant gastric juice may cause diffuse, boardlike rigidity.

Important observations concerning rigidity in the presence of abdominal injury include: (1) Rigidity may be slight, and may be either general or local. (2) It may be confined to one part or it may become diffuse, generally indicating hemorrhage or a gastro-intestinal lesion. (3) There may be alternating presence and absence of rigidity, a finding sometimes accompanied by extensive injuries. (4) The term "apprehensive rigidity" has been applied to the condition in which the abdomen looks soft and moves on respiration but becomes rigid when the hand approaches to palpate. As a rule this is accompanied by no serious injury. (5) Boardlike rigidity, with extreme pain, nearly always indicates that there is a wound of the gastro-intestinal tract. (6) Complete absence of rigidity is usually a very bad sign, when there are visceral lesions. (7) Morphine in moderate doses seems to have very little effect on tension of the abdominal wall.

Palpation for Foreign Bodies, Defects in Parietes, and Crepitation. —Palpation of the *abdominal wall,* the *lower thoracic wall,* the *buttocks,* and the *upper parts of the thighs* may reveal a missile lodged superficially, near the wound of entrance, or in a region where a wound of exit would have occurred had the projectile traveled slightly farther. Subcutaneous rupture of the abdominal wall caused by blunt force may be revealed by a *gap in a muscle.* The detection by palpation of *crepitus* due to subcutaneous emphysema, may indicate the presence of an associated thoracic wound. Crepitation occurring late may be due to gas bacillus infection. Occasionally, the diffusion of air which has been trapped beneath a flap of soft tissue, as well as diffusion into the parietal wall of gas which has escaped through a gastric perforation, is responsible for palpable crepitation in the abdominal wall. Crepitation may also sometimes be due to an intra-mural abdominal hematoma.

Rectal Examination.—Rectal examination should be performed especially when the wound of entrance is in the gluteal, sacral, or peri-neal region. Not only can perforations of the anorectal region be found, but blood on the gloved finger may disclose bleeding from a wound of the colon above the reach of the examining finger.

Examination for Residual Abscesses and for Fluid in Peritoneal Cavity.—Physical examination for residual abscesses which develop in the postoperative period, or when treatment has been conservative, includes *rectal examination* for revealing loss of tonus of the anal sphincter and the presence of masses in the pelvis due to suppuration in the rectovesical space; the *eliciting of tenderness* on pressure over the twelfth rib, which is usually possible in the presence of subphrenic infections, and the *finding of tenderness or a mass* in various regions of the abdomen, such as the iliac fossa.

Ballottement may reveal the accumulation in the peritoneal cav-ity of blood, gastro-intestinal contents or, in late cases, fluid inflamma-tory exudate.

Percussion

Percussion may show absence or diminution of relative or absolute hepatic dulness due to free gas in the peritoneal cavity. The absence of this sign, even though a gas-filled hollow viscus has been perforated, is sometimes due to the external escape of gas through the wound in the abdominal wall. Percussion may also reveal abnormal dulness in the flanks, or shifting dulness because of blood in the peritoneal cavity.

Auscultation

There is seldom occasion to auscultate the abdomens of patients with recent abdominal injury. Late after the injury, however, the detection of the so-called silent abdomen may indicate the presence of ileus or peritonitis.

Temperature

Oral, rectal, or axillary temperature in the presence of shock and hemorrhage is likely to be subnormal, sometimes as much as 2° below normal. Elevation of the temperature usually indicates peritonitis or other infection, although it may be due to extravasation of blood, either in the abdominal wall or into the peritoneal cavity.

Blood Pressure

Determinations of blood pressure are often helpful, not only in estimating the patient's initial condition but in serving as a therapeutic guide in preoperative preparation and in determining the safe time for operation. A systolic blood pressure of *80 mm. of mercury is generally accepted as the minimal level below which operation is inadvisable.* Lowering of the blood pressure is usually paralleled by a rise in pulse rate. As an indicator of the degree or continuance of hemorrhage, changes in blood pressure are, however, often undependable, because fatal hemorrhage may occur before the changes reflect the reduction of circulating blood volume. Determination of changes in the specific gravity of the blood, and estimation of the mean corpuscular volume, are more reliable methods for indicating not only the extent or progress of external or concealed hemorrhage, but also the degree of shock.

CLINICAL LABORATORY STUDIES

Examination of Urine

Examination of the urine for grossly detectable blood should be made in every case of even suspected abdominal injury. If gross blood is detected, microscopic examination of the urine may be dispensed with.

Hematologic Studies

Changes in the cellular composition and the physical properties of the blood depend not only on the rate, duration, and total volume of blood loss, but are also influenced by concomitant traumatic shock due to tissue injury and by parenteral fluid therapy. Furthermore, a degree of shock disproportionate to that which follows the external loss of a given amount of blood often occurs when the blood is spilled into the peritoneal cavity. Intraperitoneal outpouring of fluid in response to the presence of blood in the peritoneal cavity, coupled with the loss of blood fluid into the general body tissues tends to cause hemoconcentration, which may mask the actual loss of red blood cells. The loss of fluids from the blood in rapid hemorrhage usually exceeds the movement of fluids back into the blood in the effort of the organism to restore and maintain blood volume. Depending on the amount, rate, location, and duration of hemorrhage, and on the degree of traumatic shock, as well as on the amount of fluid administered parenterally, the blood of patients with abdominal injuries may be concentrated, diluted, or practically unchanged in composition.

Blood Counts and Studies of Hemoglobin

Even repeated counts of red blood cells and determinations of hemoglobin index are *not dependable* indicators of either the amount or the continuance of hemorrhage, as significant changes in them may not occur until there has been great loss of blood. Definite lowering of the erythrocyte count and of the hemoglobin index are usually paralleled, or even preceded, by clinical evidences of continued hemorrhage.

Determinations of Corpuscular Volume and Blood Specific Gravity

Accurate information concerning either concentration or dilution of the blood, associated with shock or hemorrhage, can be obtained by the *hematocrit* determination of mean corpuscular volume, and by the *falling-drop* method for estimating the specific gravity of whole blood and plasma, from which values the level of serum protein can be calculated. The following are the normal values obtained in the studies just discussed:

Cell Volume.—For males, the average cell volume is 46 per cent, with a range from 42 to 50 per cent. For females, the average is lower, being 41 per cent, with a range from 39 to 43 per cent.

Specific Gravity of Whole Blood.—The average value of peripheral blood of males is 1.0566, while that of females is 1.0533. There occurs a daily swing of 0.0033, the blood being more concentrated in the morning.

Specific Gravity of Plasma.—The average for both sexes is 1.0270, with a normal range from 1.0253 to 1.0288. The purpose of estimating this is that, in addition to giving information about plasma solids, it affords a quick, reliable method for determining plasma proteins.

Plasma Proteins.—For both males and females, there are approximately 70 gm. of proteins for each liter of plasma, with normal variations between 5.9 and 7.9 gm. per 100 cc.

Changes in the composition and physical character of the blood depend not only on the rate, duration, and total volume of blood loss, but are also influenced by concomitant traumatic shock due to tissue injury, and by parenteral fluid therapy. Blood studies following abdominal trauma therefore often reveal only slight or confusing deviations from the normal. A degree of shock disproportionate to that which follows the external loss of a given amount of blood often occurs when the blood is spilled into the peritoneal cavity. The intraperitoneal outpouring of fluid in response to the presence of the blood, coupled with the loss of blood fluid into the tissues, tends to cause hemoconcentration and this trend in the composition of the blood can mask the actual loss of red blood cells. The loss of fluids from the blood often exceeds the movement of fluids into the blood in the effort of the organism to restore and maintain blood volume. Therefore, depending on the location, amount, rate, and duration of hemorrhage, and the degree of associated traumatic shock, as well as the fluid administered parenterally, the blood of patients with abdominal injuries may be concentrated, diluted, or practically unchanged in composition.

BACTERIOLOGIC STUDIES

Examination of direct smears, or growths of anaerobic and aerobic micro-organisms, obtained on cultures made with material from the edges of wounds or from wound exudate, may help in choosing appropriate chemotherapeutic or other agents for prophylaxis or treatment of peritonitis or wound infection.

ROENTGENOLOGIC EXAMINATION

When *missiles* are retained within the abdomen or when there is a possibility that more than one projectile has entered the abdomen or the abdominal wall, roentgenoscopic or roentgenographic examinations should be done. The use of portable roentgenologic apparatus saves moving the patient on and off a table, and sometimes roentgenologic examinations are best done in the operating room. Roentgenologic examination not only yields information which is valuable in planning operative incisions in respect to retained missiles, but often reveals *gas* beneath the diaphragm, diaphragmatic *hernia,* and the *mobility* or *fixation* of the diaphragm. The absence of gas beneath the diaphragm, even though a hollow gastro-intestinal viscus has been perforated, may be due to the escape of gas through the wound in the abdominal wall.

When more than roentgenoscopic examination is necessary, anteroposterior and lateral roentgenograms usually furnish sufficient data and permit fairly accurate localization of foreign bodies. Stereoscopic roentgenograms, however, are sometimes much more valuable than a single projection. If precise localization of a foreign body is required, such information can be obtained by one of the following methods: (1) rotation of the parts; study of the movement of the shadows of the projectiles or other foreign bodies in relation to neighboring opaque structures or skin markers; (2) the "nearest point" method; (3) the parallax method, which is often combined with the "nearest point" method; (4) the orthodiagraphic method, which is often combined with the "nearest point" method; (5) the method of right angled planes (four point survey); (6) the multiple diameters method; (7) the single shift triangulation method, with which can be included the stereoscopic method; (8) the double shift, fixed angle method; (9) the harpooning method, combined with reconstruction of the part by the aid of a cross section anatomic atlas. There are numerous other methods which might be described, but those already mentioned are all simple, quickly performed and accurate to within 0.5 cm., without the aid of plates. Planographic or tomographic methods of localization are satisfactory but require special apparatus.

Roentgenographic examinations, or roentgenoscopic observations made in a darkened operating room or with the aid of a roentgenoscopic bonnet, are seldom necessary during operations for abdominal injuries. The method of intermittent roentgenoscopic control was found to be more satisfactory in the war of 1914–1918 for general use in the extraction of metallic foreign bodies than were electrovibrators, telephone probes, or other similar devices, because approximately one-fifth of the foreign bodies were not magnetizable.

Intravenous pyelo-ureterography as well as retrograde cystography is sometimes useful in determining not only the existence but the extent and complications of injuries involving the kidneys, ureters, and bladder.

Late in the postoperative period, or if patients have been treated by entirely conservative measures, roentgenologic studies are useful in revealing the presence of subphrenic residual abscesses or other intraperitoneal suppuration.

ENDOSCOPIC EXAMINATION

Endoscopic examinations are occasionally informative when other methods fail to furnish conclusive data.

Proctoscopy or *sigmoidoscopy* may disclose an injury of the terminal portion of the large bowel, either by affording visualization of a wound which is not detectable by the examining finger, or by merely revealing the presence of blood.

Esophagoscopy and *gastroscopy* may be employed when injury to the esophagus or the stomach is merely suspected. As in the instance of proctoscopic and sigmoidoscopic examinations, even though it may be impossible to see a perforation in either the esophagus or the stomach, detection of blood is of diagnostic value.

Cystoscopic examination cannot be performed satisfactorily when the bladder has been perforated because it is impossible to distend it with water. In the absence of perforation of the bladder, however, cystoscopy may permit detection of bleeding from a ureteral orifice due to either renal or ureteral injury. The preoperative introduction of a large catheter into a ureter from which bleeding has been observed, facilitates its repair after the abdomen has been opened.

PERITONEOSCOPY

This method of examination is variously known as "abdominoscopy," "celioscopy," "laparoscopy," or "ventroscopy." Although inadequate for determining definitely whether or not visceral perforation has occurred, peritoneoscopy may avert unnecessary laparotomy.

Peritoneoscopy can be performed by means of a foroblique cystoscope and simple accessories. However, the Ruddock peritoneoscope gives visibility and range far superior to the cystoscope. The peritoneoscope is introduced through a small incision and the areas of the parietal peritoneum through which perforation might possibly have occurred are surveyed. When a perforation is found, exploration should be done even though no blood, gastro-intestinal contents, bile or urine is detected, as it is not safe to depend on peritoneoscopic examination to determine whether or not visceral perforation has occurred. The following technic for peritoneoscopy is recommended: (1) After local infiltration with procaine, a small stab wound is made down to the transversalis fascia, usually in the median line just below the umbilicus. (2) While the patient makes tense his abdominal wall, a blunt spinal puncture needle is introduced into the peritoneal cavity and the abdomen is slowly distended with air. (3) Through the same stab wound, penetration is then safely completed by the trocar, which is of the same size as the sheath of the peritoneoscope. On its withdrawal, the peritoneoscope is immediately inserted and additional air, as needed, is injected through the turncock. (4) After the peritoneoscope is in place, large, curved hemostat forceps are gently introduced into the wound of entry (which has been subjected to débridement) so as to indent the underlying peritoneum. This localizes the area of suspected perforation. Shifting the viscera by appropriate tilting of the patient or displacement of viscera by an instrument introduced through the peritoneoscope often will allow visualization of regions which are otherwise inaccessible to view. Hemoperitoneum, except when obviously due to instrumentation, is in itself proof of penetration.

DETERMINATION OF PENETRATION BY EXPLORATION

Exploration of Wound

When complete penetration of the abdominal wall is in doubt, it may be possible, by means of a pair of blunt forceps used as a probe, to determine whether or not the perforation extends through the parietal peritoneum. When a wound extends obliquely for a considerable distance in the abdominal wall, however, a shift in muscle, fascia or fat may make it impossible to follow the entire tract, so that this method is not always dependable. Although the probing of wounds has been deprecated, much valuable information may be obtained safely by this simple method.

When there is uncertainty concerning perforation of the peritoneal membrane, an incision may be made down to the peritoneum near the wound of entry in the abdominal wall and then, by peeling away the peritoneum in the region of the wound, the presence or absence of peritoneal perforation usually can be determined.

Exploratory Laparotomy

When, despite the employment of various methods of determining if peritoneal perforation or visceral penetration has occurred, doubt still exists concerning such possible injuries, early exploration is usually safer than prolonged observation and conservative treatment. Because of the previous escape of gas through the wound in the abdominal wall, the hissing sound, such as is often heard when the peritoneum is opened following rupture of a peptic ulcer, is frequently absent in cases of penetrating wounds of the abdomen, even though a gas filled hollow viscus has been perforated.

Although blood, and less frequently extravasated gastro-intestinal contents, may be found as soon as the peritoneum is incised, the location of the injury may be so distant, or the amount of free fluid in the part of the abdominal cavity first brought to view may be so small that, until exploration has been carried farther, it is not possible to determine whether there has been visceral injury.

REFERENCES

1. Barbour, H. G., and Hamilton, W. F.: Blood Specific Gravity: Its Significance and a New Method for Its Determination. Am. J. Physiol. *69:* 654–661, 1924.
2. Bastos, M.: Sobre el Pronóstico en las Heridas de Guerra del Vientre. Rev. de Sanidad de Guerra. *2:* 1–17 (Jan.), 1938.
3. Granger, Amedee: II. Radiological Signs of Subdiaphragmatic Abscess. New Orleans M. and S. J. *82:* 748–751 (May), 1930.

4. Hamilton, J. E.: Peritoneoscopy in Gunshot and Stab Wounds of the Abdomen. Surgery. *7:* 582–588 (Apr.), 1940.

5. Meyer, K., and Shapiro, P. F.: Treatment of Abdominal Injuries: Collective Review. Internat. Abstr. Surg. *66:* 245–257, 1938.

6. Scudder, John: Shock: Blood Studies as a Guide to Therapy. Philadelphia, J. B. Lippincott, 1940.

7. Storck, Ambrose H.: Diagnosis in Abdominal Trauma. Am. J. Surg. *56:* 21 (April), 1942.

8. Taylor, F. W.: Gunshot Wounds of the Abdomen. J. Indiana M. A. *31:* 342–345 (July), 1938.

9. The Medical Department of the United States Army in the World War: Cited before.

10. Wallace, Cuthbert: Cited before.

11. Wright, L., Wilkinson, R. S., and Gaster, J. L.: Penetrating Stab Wounds of the Abdomen and Stab Wounds of the Abdominal Wall: Review of 184 Consecutive Cases. Surgery. *6:* 241–260 (Aug.), 1939.

12. Wrork, D. H.: A Study of Abdominal Rigidity. Proc. Staff Meet., Mayo Clin. *15:* 393–398 (June), 1940.

CHAPTER IV

GENERAL CARE OF PATIENT, INCLUDING PREOPERATIVE PREPARATION

CARE of abdominal casualties should continue without interruption during transportation and in the hospital. Immediate attention must usually consist of dusting the wound and any extruded viscera with 5 gm. of sulfanilamide or other sulfonamide drug and firmly applying a sterile dressing. Preoperative study and preparation of extremely ill patients should be made in or near the operating room, to permit immediate operation at the time of first improvement in respect to shock and hemorrhage.

TREATMENT OF SHOCK AND HEMORRHAGE

General Measures

Preservation of body heat, gentle handling, rest, and relief of pain are the simplest and the most effective methods of averting or treating shock. Patients with abdominal injury usually are most comfortable if placed so that the abdominal muscles are relaxed. The head-down position during transportation is of value in combating shock. The application of tourniquets to prevent loss of blood, as well as to prevent absorption from damaged extremities, also reduces shock. *Morphine sulfate* should be administered in doses of from ¼ to ¾ grain (0.016 to 0.05 gm.), depending on the size of the patient and the extent of the injury. The effectiveness of treatment for shock is in large measure determined by the promptness with which it is instituted.

Transfusion of Whole Blood and Blood Elements

Blood plasma is superior to other fluids for overcoming hemoconcentration associated with shock, unless shock is due to severe hemorrhage, when fresh or preserved *whole blood* is preferable. Good results in treatment of shock with pituitary extract and concentrated plasma or serum have been reported. *Concentrated serum albumin* probably will be of limited usefulness in treatment of abdominal cas-

37

ualities. There is danger of increased or renewed hemorrhage due to the rise in blood pressure which follows its use but patients with abdominal wounds should not take water by mouth.

In massive or continuing hemorrhage large amounts of whole blood or liquid blood elements, or even continuous transfusion, may be desirable. Transfusion of as much as 3000 cc. within a few hours may be required. In addition to clinical methods for deciding on the need for transfusion, determinations of mean corpuscular volume and studies of blood specific gravity furnish even more accurate information.

Plasma and whole blood are equally effective for restoring blood volume, and if transfusion is to be large, only 1 pint (about 500 cc.) in each 3 pints (about 1500 cc.) of plasma and blood need be whole blood. In secondary shock, a rise of from 10 to 20 mm. of mercury usually can be anticipated from every 500 cc. (approx.) of blood transfused, if bleeding has ceased and no other causes of loss of circulatory fluid exist. Differentiation is to be made between (1) primary shock, due to psychogenic and neurogenic influences, from which recovery rapidly occurs following rest and administration of morphine, and (2) secondary shock, which is indicated by persistence of low systolic blood pressure (less than 100 mm. of mercury) even after one hour of treatment by simple measures, and in which transfusion is necessary. Practically complete replacement of lost fluid is required, and at least half of this should be protein fluid, as otherwise restoration of blood pressure will be only temporary.

Infusions

When supplies of liquid or dried blood elements or of whole blood are not available, it may be necessary to give infusions of 5 per cent *solution of glucose*, either alone or with *physiologic saline or lactated Ringer's solution*, even though such solutions rapidly pass out of the vascular tree and usually fail to sustain blood volume.

Although rapid intravenous administration of large amounts of fluids may raise the blood pressure sufficiently to increase or renew hemorrhage, long sustained severe hypotension will cause death, so early restitution of blood volume must be accomplished by slow infusions or transfusions.

Since even large infusions may be safely administered intravenously, using fluids either at room temperature or after recent removal from a refrigerator, elaborate apparatus for warming the solutions or keeping them at body temperature is unnecessary. Since solutions of glucose of a concentration of more than 5 per cent are likely to produce ileus, they should be buffered with insulin, in the proportion of 1 unit of insulin to each 2.5 gm. of glucose in excess of the amount necessary to make a 5 per cent solution.

Mobile Unit for Study and Treatment of Shock and Hemorrhage

Mobile equipment for the study and treatment of shock and hemorrhage at the bedside or in the operating room should include the

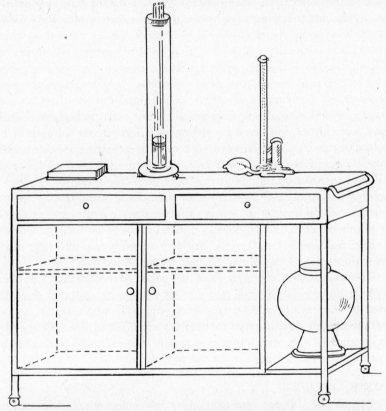

Fig. 9.—Portable "shock cart" which includes apparatus and supplies for studying and treating shock and hemorrhage. Indicated on top are pieces of apparatus for falling-drop estimations, blood-cell counts, and determinations of blood pressure. The centrifuge is for studies of mean corpuscular volume. The drawers contain syringes, sterile linen, and direct transfusion equipment. The compartments below contain plasma, whole blood, saline and glucose solutions, tubing, drip meters, and drugs.

following: (a) falling drop apparatus; (b) centrifuge for determination of the mean corpuscular volume; (c) sphygmomanometer; (d) blood counting and hemoglobin index equipment; (e) supplies of

preserved or whole blood, serum or pooled plasma; (f) blood match-
ing materials and direct transfusion apparatus, and (g) supplies of
glucose and lactated Ringer's solution. Such a mobile "shock cart"
should also contain blankets, hot water bags and blocks for elevating
the foot of the bed (Fig. 9).

Drug Therapy for Shock and Hemorrhage

The administration of *epinephrine, ephedrine,* or *pituitary extract*
can, by suddenly raising blood pressure, increase or reinstitute bleeding. Following the brief elevation of blood pressure caused by these
drugs, there is usually a fall, often to a level below that which existed
beforehand. Nevertheless, when the blood pressure is extremely low,
administration of these drugs, or of *caffeine sodiobenzoate, pentamethylenetetrazol* (*metrazol*), or 25 per cent solution of pyridine betacarboxylic acid diethylamide (*coramine*), may seem necessary. Suprarenal cortical hormone, in conjunction with hypertonic solution of sodium chloride has been advocated for the treatment of shock on the
basis that suppression of secretion of suprarenal cortical hormone
with loss of isosmotic fluids of the blood into the interstitial spaces is
thereby counteracted. Preparations containing suprarenal cortical
hormone, or the synthetic desoxycorticosterone acetate, are available
for administration intravenously, intramuscularly or subcutaneously,
usually in doses of 1 to 2 mg. every four to six hours, although much
larger doses have been given without undesirable effects.

Treatment with digitalis is of no value in combating the sinus
tachycardia associated with penetrating wounds of the abdomen. Instead of increasing cardiac efficiency, digitalis administered to patients wounded thus impairs cardiac function, for in the absence of a
disturbance of the conduction mechanism, the only effect exerted by
digitalis is its toxic influence on the myocardium.

Oxygen Therapy

The use of 100 per cent oxygen by inhalation is an additional effective method of treating shock. If special oxygen equipment is not
available, the nasal catheter method can be employed to increase
alveolar oxygen tension.

PREOPERATIVE ANTITOXIN THERAPY

If the patient has been previously immunized by means of tetanus
toxoid, a *stimulating dose of toxoid* should be given. If he has not previously been immunized, a dose of *3000 units of tetanus antitoxin*
should be given subcutaneously immediately after injury, as well

as preceding any subsequent operation. In the presence of *seriously contaminated* wounds it is sometimes advisable to administer also *polyvalent serum,* which contains antibodies against Bacillus perfringens (Clostridium welchii), Vibrion septique (Clostridium oedematis maligni), Bacillus haemolyticus (Clostridium haemolyticum), and Bacillus oedematiens (Clostridium oedematiens). Antiserums should be given shortly following admission of the patient to the hospital unit, after the absence of serum sensitivity has been determined or, if necessary, after desensitization. The protection against anaphylactic reactions afforded by ether and other general anesthetic agents may be taken advantage of by administering antiserums while the patient is anesthetized.

REFERENCES

1. Best, C. H., and Solandt, D. Y.: Use of Plasma or Serum as a Substitute for Whole Blood. Brit. M. J. 2: 116–117 (July), 1940.
2. Boothby, W. M., Mayo, C. W., and Lovelace, W. R., II.: The Use of Oxygen and Oxygen-helium, with Special Reference to Surgery. S. Clin. North America. 20: 1107–1168 (Aug.), 1940.
3. Harkins, H. N.: Cited before.
4. Kekwick, A., Marriott, H. L., Maycock, W. d'A., and Whitby, L. E. H.: Cited before.
5. Ochsner, Alton, and Cutting. R. A.: Effect of Insulin and Glucose in Normal and Obstructed Intestine. Proc. Soc. Exper. Biol. and Med. 29: 264–265 (Nov.), 1931.
6. Scudder, John: Cited before.
7. Storck, Ambrose H.: Cited before.
8. The Medical Department of the United States Army in the World War: Cited before.
9. Wallace, Cuthbert: Cited before.

CHAPTER V

SELECTION OF PATIENTS FOR OPERATION

PATIENTS DEFINITELY REQUIRING OPERATION

CELIOTOMY usually should be performed immediately when there is known or suspected visceral injury of recent occurrence, not associated with severe shock or extensive injuries to other parts, but there are exceptions to this general rule (Fig. 10).

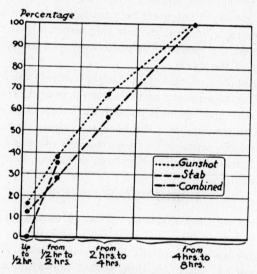

Fig. 10.—Curve indicating the mortality in relation to the period elapsed from the time of admission at hospital to the time of operation, in forty-six cases of penetrating wound of the abdomen. The form of this curve is, in part, due to the good condition of those patients on whom early operation could be performed without prolonged preoperative preparation.

PATIENTS IN HOPELESS CONDITION

When an abdominal injury is of long duration, or is so extensive that satisfactory anatomic repair or functional restitution is evidently impossible, operation not only unnecessarily subjects the patient to added discomfort, but consumes time and materials which might be employed to better advantage in caring for patients who have a chance of recovery.

PATIENTS NOT REQUIRING OPERATION

In contrast with the cases in which operation is definitely indicated, and with those in which the factor of time or the extent of the injury makes operation seem hopeless, are those in which even exploration of the abdomen seems unnecessary because it is considered that the injury will not prove fatal. Elective nonoperative management is most often warranted when the injury is limited to the *upper part of the abdomen,* especially to the region of the *liver,* and particularly if the injury has been caused by a small projectile. Due to continued hemorrhage or the retention of projectiles, operative intervention may be required in some of these cases. Less frequently than in the instance of wounds involving the region of the liver, nonoperative management must be considered when there is a *high abdominothoracic wound on the left side,* especially if the projectile has entered near the median line posteriorly and has emerged in the posterior part of the axilla.

The advisability of operation cannot entirely be based on the location, size, or appearance of the external wound or on the size of the missile. Although wounds caused by small missiles, especially those limited to the region of the liver, sometimes do not require exploratory celiotomy, apparently trivial wounds often are accompanied by extensive intraperitoneal hemorrhage or gaping, lacerated wounds of hollow viscera.

BORDERLINE CASES

Patients who do not reach an operating unit until *twelve hours* or longer after injury constitute poor risks regardless of the extent of the injury, and operation usually only hastens death. Fibrinous exudate or edema has often by then sealed perforations of a hollow viscus. Even after *six hours,* protective barriers are fairly well established and operative manipulation results in the breaking down of natural defense mechanisms. When wounds involve only the *upper part of the abdomen,* the period during which operation is warranted is *longer,* not only because continued hemorrhage from the liver or spleen may demand operation, but because the frequent absence of hollow visceral perforations in such cases makes late operation relatively safe. Due to the irreversible deleterious effects of prolonged shock, rapid preparation for operation should always be attempted, but sometimes intentional delay of operation for several hours may be necessary for adequate preparation. When it is impossible to improve the patient's condition as much as might be desired, celiotomy must at times be performed, even though there has been only partial recovery from shock. When there is little initial shock, operation should be done promptly to avert possible development of shock due to continuous slight bleeding, subsequent massive hemorrhage, or other causes.

CHAPTER VI

PREANESTHETIC PREPARATION AND ANESTHESIA

PREANESTHETIC PREPARATION

IF *morphine* has been given within two hours or less before anesthesia is begun, an additional dose as a part of preanesthetic preparation is unnecessary. In addition to its respiratory stimulating effect *scopolamine* causes less thickening of bronchial secretions than does *atropine*. Preanesthetic sedation by oral administration of derivatives of *barbituric acid,* such as pentobarbital sodium (nembutal) or sodium propylmethylcarbinylallylbarbiturate (seconal), in doses of 3 grains (0.2 gm.) as used in the preparation of patients for elective surgical procedures, is frequently either impossible or undesirable in cases of abdominal injury. Anesthesia can be induced, however, by intravenous injection of a 5 per cent solution of pentothal sodium. The administration of barbiturates to patients who are to be anesthetized with cyclopropane has been condemned on the basis that such a sequence results in a high incidence of laryngospasm.

When operation must be immediately performed, $\frac{1}{6}$ grain (0.01 gm.) of *morphine sulfate,* and $\frac{1}{100}$ grain (0.00065 gm.) of *atropine sulfate* may be administered intravenously in 10 cc. of sterile water or physiologic saline solution.

ANESTHESIA

Choice of the anesthetic agent is based on the patient's condition in respect to shock and hemorrhage, on the existence of thoracic or other associated extra-abdominal injuries and on the extent of the operative procedure estimated to be necessary.

Spinal Anesthesia

Spinal anesthesia offers distinct advantages in many cases in which shock and hemorrhage are not pronounced. Table 1, which indicates the various types of anesthesia used in a series of cases in which penetrating wounds of the abdomen were present, shows that contrary to the frequently expressed opinion, this type of anesthesia may at times safely be employed.

Recent improvements in continuous spinal anesthesia suggest that this method may be applicable in some cases of abdominal injury.

Contraindications to Spinal Anesthesia.—There are three contraindications to spinal anesthesia for patients who have abdominal wounds. The *first* is extreme shock. The systolic blood pressure must not be less than 90 mm. of mercury and the pulse pressure not less than half the diastolic pressure. The pulse rate must not be more than 120 beats per minute; the respiratory rate not more than 30 per minute and, because respiratory depression frequently follows, spinal anes-

TABLE 1.—MORTALITY IN RELATION TO ANESTHESIA IN A SERIES OF 46 PENE-
TRATING WOUNDS OF ABDOMEN

		Anesthetic Agent or Method						
		Ether	Eth-ylene	Spinal and Eth-ylene	Spinal and Ether	Spinal	Local	Local and Ether
Gunshot	Lived	10	2	1	1	6	0	1
	Died	13	0	0	0	0	1	0
Stab	Lived	1	1	0	0	4	2	0
	Died	1	1	0	0	0	1	0
Combined	Lived	11	3	1	1	10	2	1
	Died	14	1	0	0	0	2	0

thesia should not be used if cyanosis is present. The *second* contraindication is associated injury to the spinal column or spinal cord. The *third* is encountered when conditions exist in which the patient cannot conveniently be turned or manipulated into a position in which spinal puncture can be done.

Peridural Anesthesia

Peridural (epidural) anesthesia, while having some of the good features of intrathecal spinal anesthesia, is less reliable than the latter. In addition to the frequently delayed action of peridural anesthesia, another objection to it is that lowering of blood pressure may be as extreme as that which sometimes follows ordinary spinal anesthesia.

Local Anesthesia

Local anesthesia is time-consuming and *generally unsatisfactory* for patients who require considerable exploration or repair of extensive injuries, but if shock or associated thoracic injuries make other types of anesthesia hazardous, then regional block anesthesia must be employed. Infiltration of the lower intercostal nerves with procaine solution can be employed to facilitate closure of wounds, especially those in the upper part of the abdomen, when the degree of relaxation afforded by inhalation anesthesia is insufficient.

Inhalation Anesthesia

The general availability and relative safety of *ether* and the simplicity of its administration probably will continue to make this a frequently chosen anesthetic agent. The high concentration of oxygen which can be maintained in the anesthetic mixture when *cyclopropane* or *ethylene* gas anesthesia is employed, makes these forms of analgesia particularly desirable in some cases, even though they produce poor relaxation. The explosiveness of cyclopropane and ethylene when mixed with oxygen, to some extent limits their usefulness. The anoxemia, which must necessarily be maintained when *nitrous oxide* is employed as the anesthetic agent, makes this gas unsatisfactory. *Vinethene,* although suitable as an anesthetic agent for operative procedures on the abdominal wall, is inadequate when intraperitoneal exploration or repair is necessary.

When there are associated thoracic wounds, inhalation anesthesia *under positive pressure* may be required. Selective intubation of a main stem bronchus may be necessary to keep only one lung expanded under positive pressure when a bronchopleural opening exists.

Intravenous Anesthesia

Intravenous administration of one of the preparations of barbituric acid, such as pentothal sodium in 5 per cent solution, is often efficient in producing muscular relaxation when this is unattainable by inhalation or regional anesthesia alone. Rarely, anesthesia can be maintained by the continued intravenous administration of 5 per cent pentothal sodium solution alone. Because of the anoxemia which is likely to accompany intravenous anesthesia, a free airway must be maintained, and administration of 100 per cent oxygen may be necessary.

REFERENCES

1. Adriani, John: Personal communication to the author.
2. Beck, M. C.: Personal communication to the author.
3. Storck, Ambrose H.: Cited before.
4. Waters, R. M.: A Study of Morphine, Scopolamine and Atropine and Their Relation to Preoperative Medication and Pain Relief. Texas State J. Med. *34:* 304–305 (Aug.), 1938.

CHAPTER VII

OPERATIVE PROCEDURE

ATTENTION TO PATIENT DURING OPERATION

SINCE the patient's general condition in respect to shock and hemorrhage is essentially the same during operation as it was immediately before, it is almost always necessary to continue treatment for these conditions during the operative procedure.

To avoid *chilling,* the temperature in the operating room should be maintained at about 75° F. and the covering of the operating table should be warmed. A blanket usually should be included in the coverings but overheating and consequent loss of fluids by sweating is to be avoided. Unnecessary exposure of the surface of the body, as well as of the viscera, should be avoided.

Comfortable placing, cushioning, and *bracing* of the patient by means of straps of adhesive plaster, special attachments to the operating table, or sand bags, not only maintain the desired position during operation but, in operations under local or spinal anesthesia, relieve the patient of the effort of trying to keep himself in the proper position. *Semiflexion* of the knees and hips, either by pillows placed under the knees or by flexing the operating table, not only affords comfort during local or spinal anesthesia but, even when general anesthesia is to be administered, such a position usually makes the patient more comfortable during the time which elapses before administration of the anesthetic agent is started, as well as following operation. In anticipation of the usual need for an infusion or transfusion, an *arm* should be placed on a board extending at a right angle from the operating table, or a *foot* should be kept accessible for this purpose. When considerable shock still exists, the *head-down* position, with support furnished by shoulder braces, is advisable. Keeping the patient in the head-down position also reduces the chance of aspiration of vomitus and facilitates removal of mucus from the air passages. When there are associated *thoracic injuries,* the *head-down* position usually should be *avoided.* In addition to observations of *pulse, respiration, blood pressure,* and *color* during operation, determinations of *mean corpuscular volume* and *specific gravity* of the *blood* are valuable indicators in respect to shock.

The *transfusion* of blood or blood elements, or the intravenous *infusion* of saline or glucose solution is almost always necessary during and after operation. Autotransfusion of blood recovered from the peritoneal cavity, or even from the thoracic cavity, is usually unsafe, because of the danger of contamination. Administration of *oxygen* alone, or the maintenance of a high percentage of oxygen in the anesthetic mixture, is effective in combating shock during operation. The unavailability of the more satisfactory methods for combating shock and compensating for loss of blood, or the persistently poor condition of the patient despite such measures, sometimes makes the use of stimulant drugs necessary.

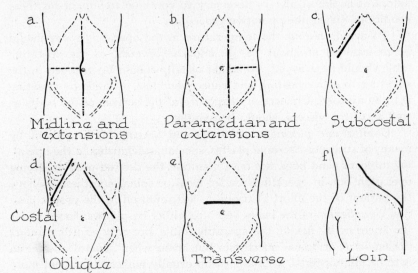

Fig. 11.—Types of incisions which can be used in cases of abdominal injury. In most cases, a midline or paramedian incision, enlarged if necessary as indicated by the dotted lines, will be most useful. Details of the costal incision represented in *d* are shown in Fig. 12. Other incisions and types of exposure, to be employed in cases of abdominothoracic injury, are shown in Figs. 42, 43, 44, and 45. The incisions which afford the best approach to the subphrenic spaces are shown in Figs. 48 and 49.

TYPES OF INCISION

Unless the abdominal wound has been caused by blunt force, the location and type of the operative incision usually is determined by the site of the wound of entry or exit, or by the position of a retained object which either can be palpated or detected by roentgenologic examination. Whenever an incision is found to be inadequate, it should be immediately enlarged or a new incision made (Fig. 11).

Vertical Incisions

Even when there is uncertainty concerning the probable location of visceral injuries, a sufficiently long and appropriately placed *midline* incision, or a *paramedian* incision is usually the best, even though a *transverse or an oblique extension* may subsequently be necessary. The division of nerves is undesirable, but an attempt to preserve them should not be allowed to interfere with rapid and adequate exposure.

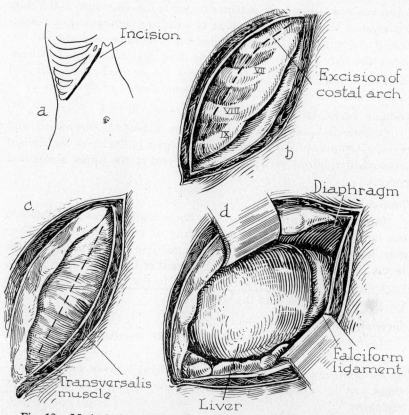

Fig. 12.—Method of resecting the costal arch to permit additional exposure of the dome of the liver. This same type of approach can be used on the left side for gaining access to the splenic flexure of the colon.

Subcostal Incisions

In the presence of in and out anteroposterior wounds in the upper right or left abdominal quadrants, an *oblique subcostal* incision may afford very good exposure, while at the same time minimizing the amount of chilling, but such incisions are often inadequate in managing the injuries encountered in military practice. A type of incision which even exposes the usually inaccessible dome of the liver is made as follows (Fig. 12): A *curvilinear* incision is made parallel to, and exposing, the sixth, seventh, eighth, ninth, and tenth costal cartilages, including the region of their fusion. These costal cartilages, or the corresponding ribs near the costochondral junctions, are then sectioned and the costal arch removed, the scalpel being kept close to the deep surface of the cartilages of the ends of the ribs. The exposed transversalis muscle is then divided in the same line as the skin. Removal of the connecting bridge of cartilage permits better retraction of the upper part of the wound and facilitates exposure of the upper and right lateral surfaces of the liver. A similar type of incision can be made on the left side to expose the stomach, the lower end of the esophagus, the spleen, or the splenic flexure of the colon.

Oblique Incisions

Oblique incisions of various lengths, extending downward and outward at appropriate angles from the region of the tip of the xiphoid process, often afford very satisfactory access to the upper abdominal regions.

Transverse Incisions

Incisions extending more or less *horizontally* across the abdomen can be used for exposing the ascending or descending colon. They may require enlargement by vertical incision of the sheath of the rectus abdominis muscle and displacement of the rectus muscle. This type of incision also may permit access to the splenic flexure of the colon, to the kidneys or to the spleen.

Incisions in Loin

Incisions such as are ordinarily used in elective surgical procedures on the urinary tract can be made either as entirely new incisions or as enlargements of existing wounds. This type of incision sometimes can be employed in exploring posterolateral wounds of the abdomen.

Miscellaneous Incisions

Depending on the location of wounds, or because of the patient's general condition, a variety of incisions in addition to those described can be extemporized. In some cases of abdominothoracic injury, especially when located on the left side, exploration of the stomach and lower end of the esophagus can be made through existing or enlarged wounds of the thoracic wall and the diaphragm. In such cases the diaphragmatic wound can be closed transpleurally.

ORDER OF OPERATIVE PROCEDURE

Treatment of Wounds of Back

Wounds situated on the back, buttocks or posterior aspect of the lower extremities should be rapidly treated before the abdomen has been opened, unless extensive intraperitoneal hemorrhage makes immediate laparotomy necessary.

Location of Bleeding Points and Arrest of Hemorrhage

As soon as the abdomen has been opened, arrest of hemorrhage should be undertaken *first*, not only to prevent additional shock, but

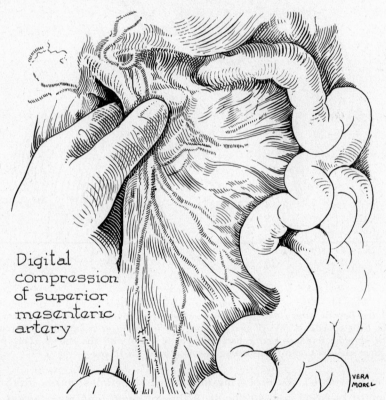

Digital
compression
of superior
mesenteric
artery

Fig. 13.—Method of digitally compressing the superior mesenteric artery. This method of temporary hemostasis may facilitate exposure and ligation of a mesenteric blood vessel which is surrounded by an obscuring hematoma.

also to eliminate interference with operative procedures caused by blood clots and liquid blood. On opening the abdomen, a degree of active hemorrhage is frequently observed which could not have existed for any length of time without having caused exsanguination. The dislocation of clots between hepatic lacerations, caused by labored breathing resulting from anesthesia, sometimes increases hepatic bleeding. The contraction of abdominal muscles, before they are relaxed by anesthesia and before laparotomy is performed, is also probably a factor in the control of bleeding from the liver.

It is usually necessary to lift out blood clots and remove liquid blood by means of suction apparatus before the source of hemorrhage

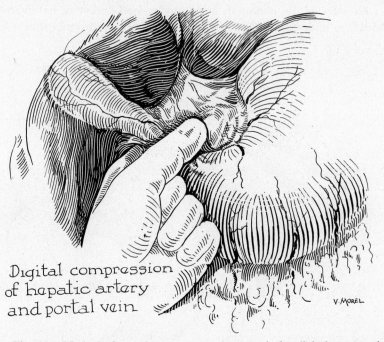

Digital compression
of hepatic artery
and portal vein

V. MOREL

Fig. 14.—Method of securing temporary hemostasis by digital compression of the hepatic artery and portal vein where they course between the layers of the hepatoduodenal fold of peritoneum. The index finger is introduced through the epiploic foramen, and counterpressure is made with the thumb. This procedure may be useful for arresting bleeding from the liver.

can be located. An obscuring hematoma sometimes makes localization of bleeding points difficult. Although much time may be lost in revealing the source of bleeding, an attempt to secure hemostasis by blindly applying clamps or introducing hemostatic sutures is dangerous. If accessible, the blood vessels supplying the region in which the hematoma is located should be digitally compressed while the hematoma is opened, evacuated, and the sources of bleeding accurately ligated. *Digital compression* of the more important blood vessels may also be employed for controlling the blood supply to regions from which bleeding for even a short time can prove fatal (Figs. 13, 14).

When there is active bleeding from the liver, the hepatic artery and portal vein may be digitally compressed, or the placing of *gauze packs* may be expedient either as a means of temporarily arresting bleeding or as a permanent method of hemostasis. The topical application of *thrombin* is an additional method of rapidly arresting serious hepatic hemorrhage.

Location and Repair of Injuries

After hemorrhage has been controlled, examination should be made of all regions or organs which are even remotely likely to have been injured. Wounds most often *overlooked* are those located at the junction of the mesentery with the small intestine; along the curvatures of the stomach; on the posterior surface of the stomach, transverse colon, rectum, or pelvic portion of the colon; in the region of the splenic flexure or hepatic flexure; and wounds of the duodenum. It is often difficult to determine with certainty the presence or absence of wounds of the liver, kidneys, or spleen unless there is active bleeding from the upper left or upper right abdominal quadrants, or unless a laceration can be felt.

Injury of the small intestine is so frequent in penetrating wounds of the abdomen that serial examination of the *entire* small bowel should be made except when the chance of such injury is extremely remote. Depending on the location of the incision, it may be best to begin examination of the small intestine at the duodenojejunal junction and proceed downward, or to start at the ileocecal junction and proceed upward.

CLEANSING OF PERITONEAL CAVITY, PERITONEAL LAVAGE, INTRAPERITONEAL INSTILLATION OF BACTERIOSTATIC SUBSTANCES

Cleansing of Peritoneal Cavity

Before closing the peritoneum, particles of feces, detached parts of viscera, accessible projectiles or fragments of projectiles, pieces of clothing, fragments of bone, or any other foreign bodies, as well as liquid or clotted blood, should be removed. As a rule, a missile should be removed only if this can be done easily, or if failure to remove it may endanger life. Unless done within *six to twelve hours*, removal of foreign bodies usually should be delayed for *six weeks* or longer.

Lavage of Peritoneal Cavity

Lavage of the contaminated peritoneal cavity with large quantities of physiologic saline solution is not only futile but *undesirable*. If there has been only localized extravasation of intestinal contents, lavage causes disseminated contamination. Furthermore, the procedure necessitates manipulation, exposure, and chilling of the intestine, and increases shock.

Intraperitoneal Instillation of Bacteriostatic Substances

The possibility of preventing or of reducing the severity of peritonitis by introducing sulfonamide drugs, either in solution or in crystalline form, into the peritoneal cavity has been the subject of many recent reports. When sulfanilamide is introduced into the peritoneal cavity the drug is absorbed so rapidly by either the normal or only recently contaminated peritoneum that its primarily local effect is probably of no more than one or two hours' duration, while at the same time such rapid absorption is likely to cause hepatic necrosis and undesirably high concentrations of the drug in the blood. For this reason only relatively small amounts, that is, not more than 10 gm., should be used when contamination has been so recent that there is not sufficient peritoneal exudate to avert undesirably rapid absorption. Doses of as much as 12 gm., when used in cases of complicated appendicitis, have been followed by no toxic effects even though the peritoneal concentrations were as high as 600 mg. per 100 cc., thirty-six hours after operation. In these same cases the drug disappeared from the blood only after 200 hours. Other sulfonamide drugs, as well as such bacteriostatic substances as penicillin and gramicidin, may in time prove even more effective than sulfanilamide in preventing peritonitis.

DRAINAGE OF PERITONEAL CAVITY

Drainage of the entire peritoneal cavity is impossible regardless of the type, number, or location of the drains, and the danger of postoperative intestinal obstruction and intestinal fistulas is increased by the presence of drains. The draining of wounds of the abdominal wall is discussed in this chapter, page 64, and the draining of localized residual abscesses is considered in Chapter X, page 121.

DÉBRIDEMENT AND ÉPLUCHAGE OF WOUNDS

Intraperitoneal injuries often so completely absorb the attention of the surgeon that wounds of the abdominal wall are either entirely neglected or inadequately treated, with resulting serious complications.

Unless treatment of wounds of the abdominal wall must be delayed because of shock, the wound should, if necessary, be *enlarged* to permit exploration. Pieces of clothing, earth, grass, gravel, splinters of wood, retained projectiles or fragments of projectiles, fragments of bone, particles of feces, loose pieces of skin, or other foreign bodies should be removed by picking them out with forceps or gently sponging them away with gauze. Since wool clothes frequently contain Bacillus perfringens (Clostridium welchii) spores, particular care must be taken to remove this possible source of gas bacillus infection. Lavage of the wound with fluids injected under enough pressure or in such a direction as to wash foreign material or loose pieces of tissue into the peritoneal cavity must be avoided.

After all loose particles have been removed from the wound, the skin, fat, fascia, muscle and strands of peritoneum which have been traumatized or deprived of their blood supply should be *cut away*. Whenever possible, removal of devitalized tissue should be done en masse, the incision being made through surrounding normal tissue, 1 cm. or more from the edge of the damaged portion. When such complete excision is thought to be unwarranted, the edges of the wound can be excised by cutting away damaged tissue from the exposed surfaces and removing undermined skin and subcutaneous tissue, so that a *beveled* edge exists about the margin of the wound. Beveling of the edges of a wound is especially important in the treatment of established infections due to aerobic or facultative aerobic organisms such as the micro-aerophilic hemolytic streptococcus. Approximation of the edges of a wound following épluchage may be impossible because of loss of tissue, or complete primary closure may be inadvisable either because of the long time that has elapsed since injury or because of the character of the material with which the wound has been contaminated.

CLOSURE OF ABDOMINAL INCISIONS INCLUDING TREATMENT, DRAINAGE, AND DRESSING OF WOUND

Closure of Abdominal Incisions

Use of Nonabsorbable Sutures and Ligatures.—The reaction caused in either clean or contaminated wounds by nonabsorbable material is so slight that wound infection and disruption are less frequent than when catgut is employed for sutures and ligatures. Although persistent sinuses sometimes follow the use of nonabsorbable material, this is

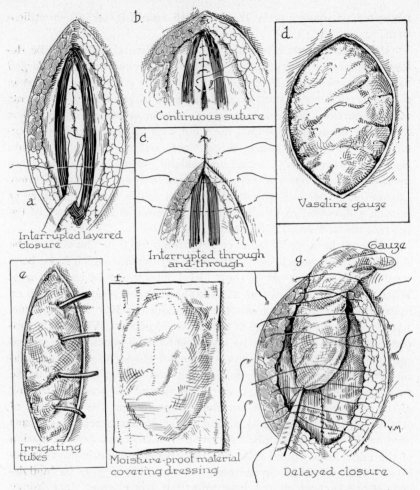

Fig. 15.—Various methods of closing wounds and incisions. *a*, Layered closure with nonabsorbable, interrupted sutures. A rubber tissue drain is placed over the peritoneum. Another drain should be placed between the edges of the sub-cutaneous fat. *b*, The method of continuous closure which can be employed when circumstances do not permit interrupted closure. *c*, Through-and-through closure. *d*, The packing with vaseline gauze which may be advisable when the wound is contaminated or infected, or which may be necessary when the large size of the wound makes approximation of its edges impossible. *e*, A wound packed with gauze, through the meshes of which tubes extend to permit introduction of anti-septic or bacteriostatic fluids. *f*, A wound in which zinc peroxide paste has been introduced and is incorporated in gauze. A sheet of cellophane or other moisture-proof substance has been placed over the wound to prevent drying of the dressing. *g*, A method of delayed closure of a contaminated wound. After closing the perit-oneum, or the peritoneum and muscle sheath, sutures which can be used for closure of the rest of the abdominal wall are introduced but not tied. Gauze, saturated with an antiseptic or bacteriostatic solution, is packed in the wound and allowed to remain in place for from twenty-four to seventy-two hours.

of little importance compared with the maintenance of approximation of the edges of the wound. Therefore wounds of the abdominal wall, whether incurred in combat or produced surgically, should be closed by means of *cotton, silk, stainless-steel wire,* or other non-absorbable sutures. The suture or ligature material should be of the smallest size consistent with tensile requirements; it should be intro-

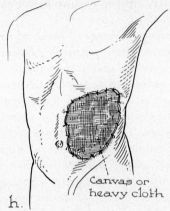

Fig. 15 (continued).—Various methods of closing wounds and incisions. *h,* How a large defect, the edges of which cannot be approximated, can be spanned with a piece of canvas or heavy cloth.

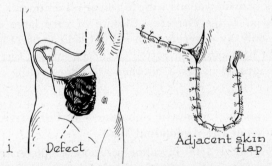

Fig. 15 (continued).—Various methods of closing wounds and incisions. *i,* The method of covering a large defect with a flap of adjacent skin.

duced in interrupted fashion, and it should be cut near the knots. Ordinarily, number 1 or number 2 braided silk is suitable for important ligations and suturing of the abdominal wall but finer silk should be used for most ligature purposes. When cotton is used, quilting cotton is preferred for closure of wounds and for important ligations. For the ligation of most bleeding points, finer cotton, number 50 or number 80, may be used.

Through-and-Through Closure.—When the necessity for *rapid closure* of the abdominal wall makes use of interrupted, layered sutures inadvisable, through-and-through or continuous closure with nonabsorbable material may be done, even though this is sometimes followed by the formation of sinuses or desmoidlike tumors of the abdominal wall. In order to prevent extension of wound suppuration to the peritoneal cavity, layered closure of the peritoneum should be done whenever possible.

Delayed or Incomplete Closure.—Delayed or incomplete closure of the abdominal wound, when *seriously contaminated,* may be done as follows: The peritoneum and transversalis fascia are closed by means of interrupted sutures of nonabsorbable material. Other sutures are then introduced, which include a loose figure of eight loop between the edges of the fascia overlying the muscles in the region, but these sutures are not tied. The wound is packed with gauze saturated with a bacteriostatic solution. After several days the packing is removed and the loosely placed sutures are then made taut and tied.

Packing of Wounds.—Vaseline gauze packing of wounds may be done either because *great loss of substance* makes closure impossible or because *contamination* of the wound makes primary closure unsafe. Favorable reports have been made on the packing of contaminated wounds with gauze which has been saturated with fish liver oil, or the filling of such wounds with fish liver oil ointment.

Covering of Large Defects.—Closure of very large defects may be possible only by covering with shifted skin flaps (Fig. 15, *i*), or by the use of light canvas or cotton cloth, cut smaller than the gaping wound and sutured in place between the edges of the wound (Fig. 15, *h*).

Antiseptic and Bacteriostatic Substances in Definitive Treatment of Wounds of the Abdominal Wall

Azochloramid, 1:3300 in saline solution, 1:500 in triacetin, and 1:1000 as an ointment, is effective in the treatment of contaminated wounds. Azochloramid is a proprietary chlorine compound containing approximately 96 per cent of N, N-dichloroazodicarbonamidine. The addition of a "wetting" solution of *sodium tetradecyl sulfate* (5 cc. to 1 liter of a 1:3300 aqueous solution of azochloramid), to lower the surface tension of the azochloramid solution, has been advocated to enhance the bactericidal properties of the azochloramid. To prevent development of infection in contaminated wounds, the direct introduction of various *sulfonamide drugs,* either crystals or powder, now appears to be of proved value. The amount of these drugs to be so used varies from 5 gm. to 10 gm., depending on the size of the wound as well as on the amount which has been either introduced into the peritoneal cavity or otherwise administered. The use of *zinc peroxide* paste in conjunction with delayed closure of wounds is efficient in combating infection caused by micro-aerophilic and anaerobic organisms.

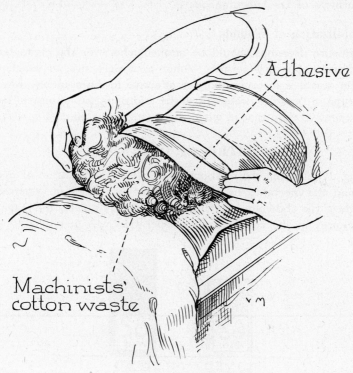

Fig. 16.—Application of pressure dressing, using machinists' cotton waste instead of marine sponges.

In addition to the antiseptic and bacteriostatic substances, such as hydrogen peroxide, which have been in common use for years, many have been developed recently but they are altogether too numerous to be individually considered.

Irrigation of Wounds

Irrigation with physiologic *saline* solution is advisable when gross contamination of the surfaces of a wound has taken place, and cleansing with *ether* is also of value.

Drainage of Wounds

Drainage of the incision of the abdominal wall usually averts the development of an intramural abscess which, should it occur and rupture into the peritoneal cavity, would cause overwhelming toxemia. *Rubber tissue drains* should be placed over the peritoneal suture line, beneath the fascia overlying the abdominal muscle, and between the cut surfaces of the subcutaneous fat.

Immobilization of Wounds

Pressure dressings should be applied whenever the character of the abdominal injury permits. Voluminous dressings, in which machinists' waste is incorporated, are effective in maintaining pressure. This type of pressure dressing has the additional advantage of being less expensive than that in which sea sponges are used (Fig. 16).

DURATION OF OPERATION

Fig. 17, showing the relationship between the duration of operation and the mortality in a series of forty-six cases of penetrating wounds of the abdomen in civil practice, in part reflects the extent of the injuries in the cases in which operation was unavoidably pro-

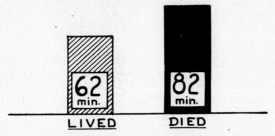

Fig. 17.—Graphic representation of the relationship between the duration of operation and the mortality in a series of forty-six cases of penetrating wounds of the abdomen.

longed. The *expediting* of operative procedures becomes imperative when large numbers of military casualties simultaneously require treatment.

REFERENCES

1. Abraham, E. P., Chain, E., Fletcher, C. M., Gardner, A. D., Heatley, N. G., Jennings, M. A., and Florey, H. W.: Further Observations on Penicillin. Lancet 2: 177–188 (Aug. 16), 1941.
2. Colebrook, Leonard: Treatment of War Wounds by Sulphonamide Packs. Lancet. 2: 113 (July 27), 1940.

3. Coller, F. A., and Valk, W. L.: The Delayed Closure of Contaminated Wounds; a Preliminary Report. Ann. Surg. *112:* 256–270 (Aug.), 1940.
4. Gage, I. M.: Gas Bacillus Infection; a Frequently Unnoticed Source in Civil Life with Report of Four cases. Am. J. Surg. *1:* 177–184 (Oct.), 1926.
5. Gordon-Taylor, Gordon: Cited before.
6. Haag, H. B., Spealman, C. R., and McCue, H. M.: Comparative Absorption Rate of Sulfanilamide from the Pleural Cavity, Peritoneal Cavity, and Gastro-intestinal Tract in Dogs. Surgery. *10:* 572 (Oct.), 1941.
7. Heilman, Dorothy and Herrell, W. E.: Mode of Action of Gramicidin. Proc. Soc. Exper. Biol. and Med. *47:* 480–484 (June), 1941.
8. Jackson, H. C., and Coller, F. A.: The Use of Sulfanilamide in the Peritoneum; Experimental and Clinical Observations. J. A. M. A. *118:* 194 (Jan. 17), 1942.
9. Meade, W. H., and Ochsner, Alton: The Relative Value of Catgut, Silk, Linen, and Cotton as Suture Materials. Surgery. *7:* 485–514 (Apr.), 1940.
10. Meleney, F. L.: Treatment of Traumatic Wounds with Zinc Peroxide. New York State J. Med. *39:* 2188–2191 (Dec.), 1939.
11. Mueller, R. S., and Thompson, J. E.: The Local Use of Sulfanilamide in the Treatment of Peritoneal Infections. J. A. M. A. *118:* 189 (Jan. 17), 1942.
12. Ogilvie, W. H.: Late Complications of Abdominal War Wounds. Lancet. *2:* 253 (Aug.), 1940; (Abstr.) War Med. (May), 1941, Vol. 1, pp. 439–442.
13. Pringle, J. H.: Notes on the Arrest of Hepatic Hemorrhage Due to Trauma. Ann. Surg. *48:* 541–549 (Oct.), 1908.
14. Shambaugh, Philip, and Dunphy, J. E.: Postoperative Wound Infections and the Use of Silk; an Experimental Study. Surgery. *1:* 379–385 (Mar.), 1937.
15. Smith, H. P.: Blood Clotting and the Control of Hemorrhage. Tr. Kansas Acad. Sc., 1937–1939, pp. 243–264.
16. Storck, Ambrose H.: Cited before.
17. The Medical Department of the United States Army in the World War: Cited before.
18. Trueta, J.: Treatment of War Wounds and Fractures with Special Reference to the Closed Method As Used in the War in Spain. New York, Paul B. Hoeber, Inc., 1940.
19. Wallace, Cuthbert: Cited before.

CHAPTER VIII

WOUNDS OF SPECIFIC STRUCTURES AND ORGANS

IN this chapter, only the signs and symptoms produced by, or the treatment peculiarly applicable to, injuries of each organ are discussed. General principles, and details of preoperative and postoperative care, are presented in Chapters IV and IX.

WOUNDS OF PERITONEUM, INCLUDING WOUNDS EXTENDING INTO PERITONEAL CAVITY, WITHOUT VISCERAL INJURY

Wounds in which a missile pierces the abdominal wall without causing visceral injury may result fatally, either because of hemorrhage due to bleeding from vessels in the abdominal wall, or because of peritonitis due to external contamination. Even though laparotomy in such cases frequently reveals no visceral injury, *exploration* is well warranted, especially if the projectile has been retained. Although, if not removed, the foreign body may become encysted and cause no subsequent symptoms, a localized peritoneal abscess often develops and requires drainage, either with or without removal of the missile.

WOUNDS OF HOLLOW ALIMENTARY ORGANS

Wounds of Esophagus

Wounds of the lower end of the esophagus are usually associated with thoracic wounds. Small injuries to the esophagus frequently are not followed either by extravasation of gastric contents or by serious hemorrhage, and they may heal spontaneously. On the other hand, the difficulty of gaining access to the lower part of the esophagus, either through the abdomen or the chest, makes the more extensive esophageal injuries exceedingly dangerous. Exposure of such wounds by an *abdominal approach* is best done through a subcostal incision, with or without division or resection of costal cartilage, or satisfactory exposure sometimes can be obtained through a left paramedian incision. Access to the esophagus is facilitated by dividing the left hepatic ligament. A piece of umbilical tape tied around the mobilized esophagus serves the triple purpose of providing a means of retraction, of preventing spilling of esophageal contents into the peritoneal cavity during operation, and of relieving tension and preventing the

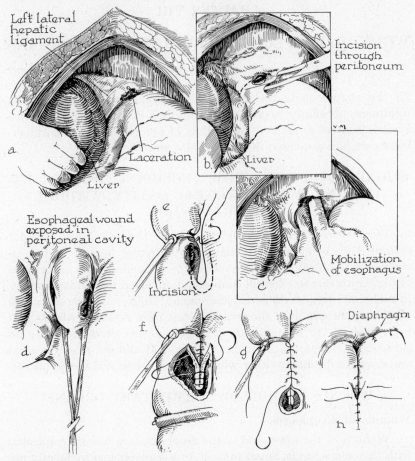

Fig. 18.—A method of exposing and repairing wounds of the esophagus. *a*, Division of the left lateral hepatic ligament and, *b*, of the peritoneum, permit exposure of the injured structure. The esophagus is mobilized, *c*, and a piece of umbilical tape, *d*, is passed around the esophagus, preventing a reflux of gastric contents. The wound is extended, *e*, and a gastro-esophageal stoma is established, *f* and *g*. Fixation of the stomach to the diaphragm, *h*, maintains relief of tension along the suture line.

tearing out of sutures which have been introduced into the thin walled and normally friable esophagus.

When there has been incomplete division of the esophagus, repair can be done by the procedure indicated in Fig. 18. When *complete division* of the esophagus has occurred, anastomosis with the cardiac end of the stomach must be attempted. This is facilitated by first incising longitudinally the esophagus, or the esophagus and the stomach, to permit formation of a sufficiently large stoma. Relaxing sutures may be introduced between the stomach and the esophagus, or between the stomach and the diaphragm, to prevent tension at the suture line. In order further to relieve tension and prevent movement in the region of the suture line, the left phrenic nerve may be crushed. For postoperative nourishing, a simple gastrostomy or jejunostomy is usually advisable. *Mediastinitis* following penetrating esophageal wounds increases the seriousness of these injuries.

Wounds of Stomach

Gastric wounds comprised about 7 per cent of all abdominal injuries among patients who came to the hospitals in the war of 1914–1918. Two-thirds of the gastric lesions were unaccompanied by other visceral injury. Other organs most frequently injured were the small intestine, liver, colon, kidney, and spleen, in the order named.

Gastric wounds are *usually two* in number, involving the anterior and posterior walls. If the anterior opening is small and the organ was not distended at the time of injury, there may be no protrusion of mucous membrane and no escape of gastric contents. If but a single wound is present, it is usually on the anterior wall. Wounds of the lesser curvature, and those parallel to the walls of the stomach, are often associated with extensive damage to the gastric wall. The posterior wall may be wounded alone, or in conjunction with the posterior surface of the transverse colon (Fig. 19). Sometimes the stomach is exposed through loss of the anterior abdominal wall, and there may even be prolapse of the stomach, accompanied by that of the colon, small bowel and spleen. Bullets which pass in an anteroposterior direction make small perforations. Shells and fragments of bombs make wounds commensurate with their size and shape. When the axis of flight of the projectile is more or less parallel to the walls of the stomach, the wounds become larger; a wound may be a linear slit, or a linear slit followed by a perforation, to which latter type of wound the term "note of exclamation wound," has been applied. The linear type of wound is nearly always on the anterior surface. When the projectile passes in through the epigastrium and out of the axilla, the slit tends to become parallel to the greater curvature. When the missile takes a more vertical course, the wounds are inclined at an angle to the greater curvature and the anterior wall or antral portion of the stomach may be almost completely divided. Projectiles striking the greater or lesser curvature in an anteroposterior direction sometimes cause rather extensive V-shaped injuries involving both walls. Occasionally, because the wound is a valvular one, escape of gastric contents is prevented. Bruises or cuts in the peritoneum or muscular coats are not infrequently found. The mucous membrane does not pout when the wounds are small, but becomes extruded in linear wounds. Hemorrhage from the wounded stomach does not as a rule occur from the gastric wall proper but from the vessels on its surface.

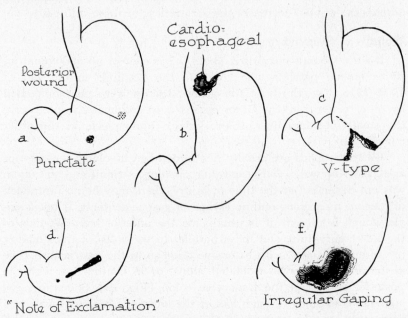

Fig. 19.—Diagrammatic representation of some common types of gastric wounds.

Symptoms Associated with Gastric Injuries.—The signs of peritoneal irritation following gastric injuries depend not only on the size and location of the wound but on the contents of the stomach. There may be signs of only *local peritoneal irritation,* or there may be diffuse *pain, tenderness,* and *rigidity. Vomiting,* including the vomiting of blood, if it occurs at all, varies greatly in amount and frequency. Hematemesis may follow concussion injuries sustained by individuals partially submerged in water near the site of explosion of a depth charge or torpedo. There is sometimes considerable *escape of gas* from the gastric wound with resulting obliteration or reduction of the normal areas of hepatic dulness.

Treatment of Gastric Injuries.—Operation should be performed in almost all cases, the only possible exceptions being those low thoracic wounds in which the stomach could have been wounded only near the esophagus or in its upper, air-containing part. A median or paramedian incision is usually best, although a subcostal incision or oblique one can be employed. Wounds on the posterior surface of the

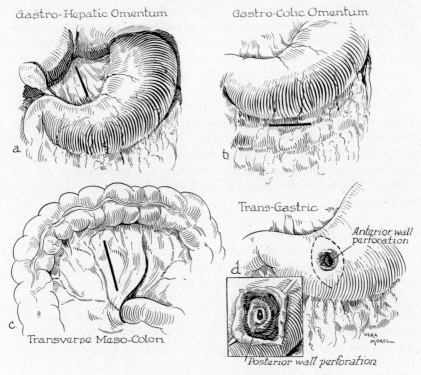

Fig. 20.—Various methods of exposing a wound of the posterior wall of the stomach: *a, b, c,* Incisions for opening the lesser peritoneal cavity; *d,* exposure of an injury of the posterior wall of the stomach through an opening in its anterior wall.

stomach can be exposed by opening the gastrohepatic omentum, the gastrocolic omentum, or the mesocolon, or by enlarging an existing wound in the anterior wall of the stomach (Fig. 20). The approach through an opening in the mesocolon, just above the transverse colon, gives good access for inspection but repair work through it is often difficult. Ragged wounds should be trimmed before suture. Gastroenterostomy is to be avoided if possible but it may be necessary when the wound divides the antral portion of the stomach or the duodenum, or when the stomach has been narrowed in the course of its repair. Performance of jejunostomy for feeding may be advisable in cases of extensive gastric wounds.

Postoperative care of gastric injuries includes the withholding of food for several days. Even limited intake of water by mouth is, as a rule, to be permitted only after establishment of suction drainage by means of a catheter extending into the stomach.

Complications of Gastric Injuries.—*Subdiaphragmatic abscess, subhepatic abscess, abscess in the lesser peritoneal sac,* and *postoperative bleeding* can follow gastric wounds. Wounds of the stomach which have been sutured, as well as those which have not been sutured, and contusions of the gastric wall may be the sites of ulceration and perforation.

Prognosis and Mortality Associated with Gastric Injuries.—Compared with injuries of the small and large intestine, gastric wounds are less serious. A favorable outcome is possible even if twenty-four to forty-eight hours have elapsed before treatment is instituted. The mortality associated with gastric wounds is approximately 55 per cent, and with uncomplicated wounds the mortality varies from 25 to 50 per cent.

Wounds of Small Intestine

Wounds of the small intestine, both complicated and uncomplicated, comprised approximately 22 per cent of all abdominal lesions in the war of 1914–1918. Associated injuries to other viscera, in the order of their frequency, are those of the colon, the stomach, the bladder, the liver, the kidneys, the rectum and the spleen. Duodenal injuries are infrequent, constituting approximately 6 per cent of all wounds of the small bowel. Injuries of the jejunum comprise about 23 per cent; and those of the ileum, approximately 71 per cent. The number of injuries in any case may vary from one to thirty, or even more, but usually there are from four to six. Injuries which can be readily sutured are more common in the upper than in the lower part of the small intestine, because of the size and thickness of the walls of the jejunum as compared with those of the ileum. The multiplicity of the coils of ileum also make it more liable to injury (Fig. 21).

Bullet Injuries of Small Intestine.—These may either open the lumen or cause only contusion or tearing of the outer intestinal coat. The *most common* injuries are perforations made by a bullet striking the intestine at a right angle to its long axis and causing two perforations, through which the mucous membrane passes out to form

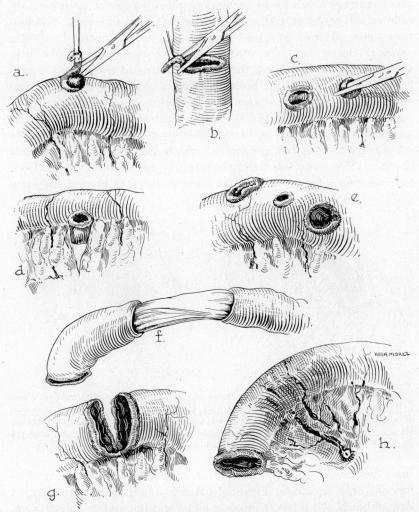

Fig. 21.—Various types of injuries of the small intestine. *a*, Single punctate wound which can be closed by a pursestring suture after removal of the everted mucosa. *b*, Simple transverse lacerated wound. *c*, Closely situated punctate wounds which can be made to communicate and then can be closed as a single wound. *d*, Wound at the junction of the mesentery with the intestine. Such wounds may be obscured by a mesenteric hematoma. *e*, Multiple punctate and lacerated wounds. In most instances such wounds should be closed individually. Resection of the bowel should be done only when separate closure of the perforations is not feasible. *f*, Injury in which the mesentery has been torn away and the muscular coats stripped back. *g*, Almost complete division of the bowel. *h*, Wound of the mesentery with thrombosis of mesenteric blood vessels and infarction of wall of bowel.

small rosettes which more or less completely prevent extravasation of intestinal contents. Owing to contraction of the intestinal musculature, some perforations appear too small to have admitted the bullet which produced them, and through such openings there may be little or no spilling, even though there is no pouting of the mucous membrane. As the flight of the bullet becomes more inclined to the transverse or long axis of the bowel, the perforations become slits. These wounds gape somewhat and the mucous membrane overlaps the cut muscular coat, so that a considerable mucous surface is seen. In other cases there is but one wound, which may involve only a small portion of the circumference of the intestine, or which may reach from the mesenteric border to a point close to the free margin. In some

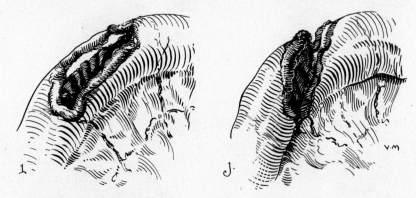

Fig. 21 (continued).—Various types of injuries of the small intestine. *i* and *j*, Extensive, lacerated wounds of the sort which sometimes necessitate resection of a small segment of intestine. The extent and character of wounds of hollow viscera caused by projectiles are determined not only by the size and shape of the missile but by the distention or collapsed state of the viscera.

cases the bowel is completely divided. In another extensive form of injury the only remaining intestinal tissue is a long, narrow and ragged strip of bowel. All types of injury may be encountered in a single case.

Injuries to Small Intestine by Fragments of Shells and Bombs.— These cause wounds of all varieties, generally commensurate with the size and shape of the projectiles. These wounds are more likely to be irregular than are those caused by bullets, and clean, transverse division of the bowel is rare.

Injuries of Small Intestine Due to Indirect Violence.—Lesions may be due to crushing blunt forces exerted through the intact abdominal wall, as well as to air and water blast wave concussion. The injuries consist in petechial hemorrhages, contusions, lacerations, and separation of the small intestine from its mesentery.

Symptoms of Injuries of Small Intestine.—*No characteristic symptoms* are associated with injuries of the small intestine. The symptoms vary with the amount of hemorrhage, the amount of spillage of intestinal contents, the coexisting wounds of other viscera, and the time elapsed since injury.

Treatment of Injuries of Small Intestine.—The point at which *exploration* of the small intestine should be begun depends on the injury and the location of the surgical wound. It may be most convenient to begin the inspection at the duodenojejunal junction, or it

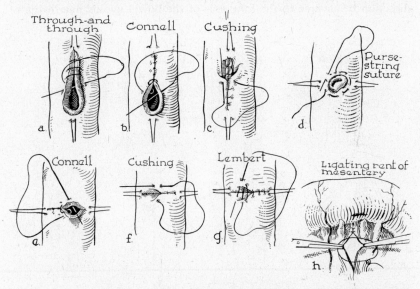

Fig. 22.—Methods of closing intestinal wounds and a method of approximating mesenteric tears. Longitudinal wounds should be closed in a transverse direction except when the wound is so long that closure in this manner would cause angulation of the bowel and greater reduction in the size of the lumen than would follow longitudinal closure. The illustrated method of approximating the edges of a lacerated or incised portion of the mesentery averts the danger of puncturing blood vessels with a needle used for introducing sutures.

may be more appropriate to begin at the ileocecal junction. A rapid survey of the bowel should be made and a careful lookout for perforations should be kept by all members of the operating team, as some of the perforations may be more readily detected from one side of the operating table than from the other. Simultaneous evisceration of the entire small intestine should be avoided, replacement of loops being done after the withdrawal of each 12 to 24 inches (about 30 to 60 cm.) of bowel. The inspection and repair of injuries to the bowel should be done so thoroughly during its first handling that subsequent inspection will not be necessary. The perforations usually should be repaired as each one is discovered. Careful search must be made at the junction of the mesentery with the intestine, for at this site a hematoma often obscures the perforation. If during the course of inspection of the small intestine a wound of the colon is seen, it can be repaired immediately in order to limit further contamination, especially if suture alone is required (Fig. 22).

Most wounds of the small intestine can be closed by means of a *single pursestring suture*. The closure of small, lacerated wounds in a direction transverse to the long axis of the bowel avoids narrowing of

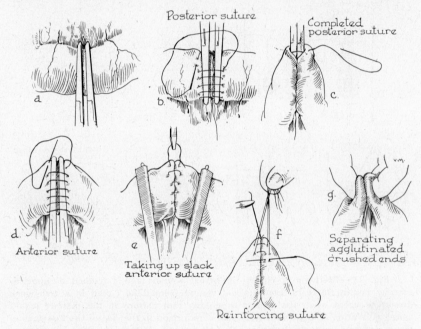

Fig. 23.—Method of end-to-end anastomosis following intestinal resection.

the lumen, but if the wound is large, this may cause angulation of the intestine at the site of repair. *Resection* should be done only when absolutely necessary, because of the high mortality associated with this procedure. The repair of a number of even closely situated wounds causes less shock than that which is produced by resection of the entire segment in which they are located. Occasionally multiple resections may be necessary, but these are rarely followed by recovery. Resection of a segment of intestine is most frequently necessary because of interference with its blood supply resulting from detachment of the bowel from its mesentery, or because of division or thrombosis of large mesenteric blood vessels. Resection also may be required when devitalization has been caused by crushing of the bowel, or when multiple wounds are in such close proximity that individual closure would reduce the size of the lumen or would cause angulation of the bowel sufficient to produce obstruction. Loss of motility and failure of the bowel to contract in response to pinching, absence of detectable pulsation in the nearby mesenteric arteries, and abnormal color of the bowel, rather than the extent of mesenteric detachment must often be depended on in determining the need for resection. An obscuring hematoma sometimes makes it impossible to ascertain the extent of injury or thrombosis of the mesenteric blood

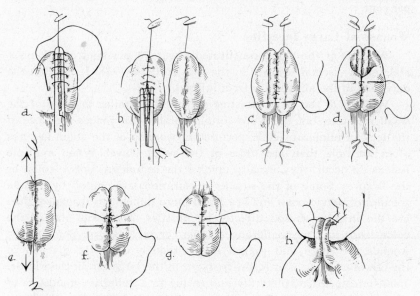

Fig. 24.—Parker-Kerr method of end-to-end anastomosis of the intestine.

vessels. When resection is done, a double row of sutures should be introduced. Devices for mechanical anastomosis, such as the Murphy button, should not be used because they may cause intestinal obstruction. End to end anastomosis is usually better than side to side anastomosis. Occasionally it is expedient to exteriorize an extensively damaged loop of small intestine or to perform an obstructive "double barrel" type of resection. A short circuiting operation, such as ileotransverse colostomy, may at times be most appropriate (Figs. 23, 24).

Although the creation of an enteric stoma at the time of operation was formerly considered to be of value as a means of averting postoperative ileus, the performance of enterostomy in anticipation of ileus has been abandoned in favor of intestinal intubation with a long or short gastro-intestinal catheter introduced through the nose.

Prognosis and Mortality Associated with Injuries of Small Intestine.—The frequency of wounds of the small intestine and the *high mortality* attending these injuries make them the major problem in military surgery of the abdomen. The mortality following wounds of the small intestine in the American Expeditionary Force in the war of 1914–1918, including the cases in which operation was performed and those in which operation was not performed, was as follows: wounds of the duodenum, 80 per cent; of the jejunum, 78.8 per cent; of the ileum, 73 per cent; part of small intestine not specified, 70.8 per cent.

Wounds of Large Intestine

Wounds of the colon constituted about 22 per cent of all intra-abdominal visceral injuries in the war of 1914–1918. It is often the only part of the alimentary tract injured.

Wounds of the large intestine are usually similar to those of the small intestine, but there are certain notable differences. Because of the lack of numerous coils, perforating wounds of the colon are less often multiple than are those of the small bowel. When multiple lesions do occur, they usually involve the redundant pelvic colon or the flexures. Some of the smaller perforations are caused by minute spicules of pelvic bone and are much more difficult to recognize than are the injuries caused directly by missiles. The large size of the colon leads to a preponderance of *tears* or *perforations*. Some of the wounds are large and ragged and, although complete division of the bowel may occur, it is less frequent in the large bowel than in the small intestine. Complete division is due to a collapsed condition of the bowel, in which state it may be only slightly larger than the small intestine. The transverse, descending and pelvic portions of the colon are the parts most frequently divided. Isolated, bruised portions of the large bowel, not infrequently remote from the tract of the missile, have been observed, while in other instances the outer coats of the large intestine have been ruptured and have retracted from the underlying intact mucosa.

Retroperitoneal perforation, with consequent fecal leakage and cellulitis, is difficult to deal with, and if the posterior perforation is a minute one, it is likely to be overlooked. Injuries of the ascending and descending portions of the colon, which have no mesenteries, are frequently followed by serious retroperitoneal infection.

Infarction of Large Intestine.—This condition, although sometimes occurring in the small intestine, is more common in the large bowel. It may result from crushing or severance of mesenteric blood vessels or it may be due to the tearing away of a segment of bowel from its mesentery.

Ulceration of Mucous Membrane of Large Intestine Associated With Rupture of Muscular Coat.—This complication may occur as soon as seven hours after wounding. It is apparently caused by cutting off of the blood supply of the mucous membrane which in turn is due to rupture of the overlying muscular coat. It has been suggested that the projectile exerts a dragging effect that is transmitted through the strands of fibrous tissue and that the damage results from this or from

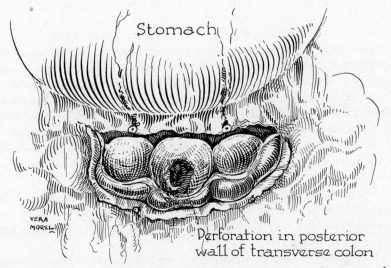

Fig. 25.—Partial mobilization and rotation of the transverse colon to reveal a perforation on its posterior aspect.

the sudden impact of the projectile on a sac filled with gas. These lesions probably account for some of the fistulas which form in cases in which the colon was thought to have escaped injury. Injuries due to air and water blast wave are likely to be of this type.

Character of Lesions in Different Parts of Colon.—Injuries of the *cecum* may be small enough to permit closure, but some are so large as to necessitate creation of an artificial anus.

Many types of wounds may involve the *transverse colon*. True anteroposterior wounds are not very common, since the transverse colon usually is struck obliquely. Wounds of the transverse colon are often accompanied by lesions of the stomach and the small intestine. The posterior surface of this segment of large intestine is sometimes

4

wounded, and injuries in this location are likely to be overlooked (Fig. 25).

The *ascending and descending* portions of the *colon* can be considered together, as neither has a mesentery. Wounds of these parts of the large intestine may be completely intraperitoneal or extraperitoneal or a combination of the two. The lesions are perforations, splits, tears or complete divisions. Perforations most commonly occur in side to side wounds, and complete divisions in anteroposterior wounds. Wounds of the ascending colon are of more frequent occurrence than those of the descending colon and the comparative rarity of wounds of the descending colon observed in the hospital is probably accounted for by the fact that this part of the colon lies so deep that a missile passing from side to side traverses a coronal plane situated so far back in the body as to involve the spinal column and great vessels. In addition, because the descending colon usually is much smaller than the ascending colon, it offers less exposed surface. The intraperitoneal wounds of the vertical colon are usually easily located and dealt with if a suitable incision has been made, but the extraperitoneal wounds, which may be small and valvular, are difficult to find because they lie in a mass of areolar tissue and may be obscured by a hematoma.

The hepatic flexure is usually easy to expose and repair because of its superficial location. Its form makes it susceptible to multiple injuries.

On account of its position and fixation, the *splenic flexure* is the most difficult part of the large intestine to examine and to repair, and mobilization of it may be necessary to permit satisfactory inspection or operative procedure.

The pelvic colon is anatomically more like the small intestine than any other part of the colon, and the lesions of the pelvic colon are somewhat similar to those of the small intestine. There may be slits, perforations, or complete divisions and, next to the injuries of the transverse colon, wounds in this segment of the large intestine are most often complicated with multiple injuries of the small bowel. The frequency of associated fracture of the pelvis increases the gravity of wounds of the pelvic colon.

Symptoms of Injuries of Large Intestine.—There may be *misleadingly few early* symptoms associated with extraperitoneal or even intraperitoneal injuries of the large intestine, especially if the latter type of wound is uncomplicated and so small that there has been little bleeding or spillage of fecal material. The appearance of patients with large wounds of the colon often resembles that caused by severe hemorrhage.

Treatment of Injuries of Large Intestine.—A *paramedian or median incision* is frequently best, because of injuries to other viscera. Such an incision is ideal for dealing with wounds of the transverse or pelvic portions of the colon. If the vertical portions of the colon or the splenic or hepatic flexure are wounded, it is sometimes necessary to supplement such an incision with a lateral extension. When the missile has only traversed the loin, and especially if a renal injury exists, a horizontal incision may be preferable, as the kidney can be dealt with through the posterior extremity of the wound. Sometimes open wounds involving the loin or iliac fossa, in which there is a possible

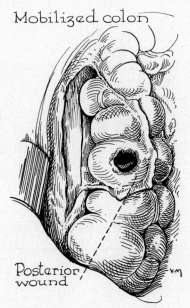

Fig. 26.—Partial mobilization and reflection of the ascending colon to reveal a retroperitoneal perforation.

injury to the colon, can be locally enlarged. The preferred incision for exposing either of the colonic flexures may be a subcostal one, prolonged vertically downward if additional space is required. This incision is especially valuable on the left side because of the posterior position and inaccessibility of the splenic angle of the colon. The oblique incision, with removal of costal cartilage, described in the section on incisions in Chapter VII, page 54, also can be employed to expose the splenic flexure. The best incision for a wound of the cecum or of the ascending or descending colon is a transverse one in the flank, for this allows easy access to the posterior portion of the bowel.

Methods of Dealing with Lesions of Large Intestine.—The general principles to be followed are: (1) *Suture* whenever possible, always employing a double row of sutures. It is often advisable to reinforce the region of repair by suturing or grafting omentum or an epiploic appendix over the suture line. (2) *Avoid immediate resection* in favor of colostomy.

In order to avoid overlooking wounds of that part of the large intestine which lacks a mesentery, the segment in which injury is suspected must be mobilized. The Trendelenburg position facilitates exposure and repair of injuries of the pelvic colon.

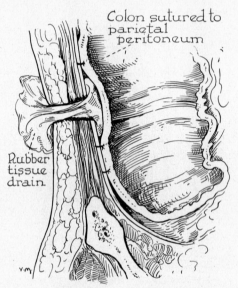

Fig. 27.—Fixation of the ascending colon and cecum to the parietal peritoneum of the lateral abdominal wall, and the introduction of a rubber tissue drain following repair of a wound in this region.

In the instance of extraperitoneal wounds which have been found only after mobilization of the colon, even though closure of the wound in the bowel is possible, it is advisable to shut off the general peritoneal cavity by a line of sutures joining the anterior surface of the bowel to the lateral abdominal wall, and to provide drainage. In the presence of hematomas it is often impossible to determine definitely the absence of colonic injuries; the region of possible injury, therefore, must be freely drained (Figs. 26, 27).

Proximal colostomy, to be of benefit, must be complete; it is most useful in the presence of wounds in the left loin, in which sepsis develops late, and in connection with rectal injuries. It may be used in

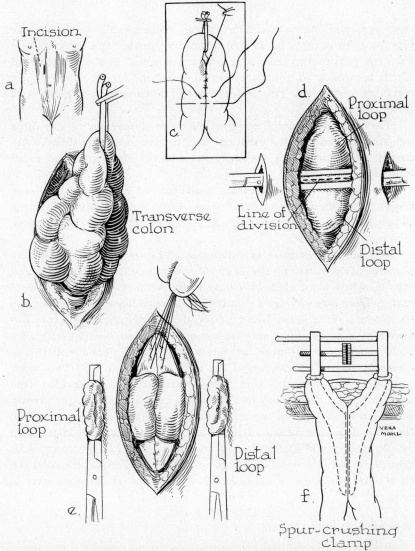

Fig. 28.—Stages in the performance of the Devine type of colostomy. This procedure can be employed also following resection of the small intestine. Its advantages are that it results in complete defunctionalization of the distal portion of the bowel and facilitates subsequent reestablishment of the continuity of the intestinal lumen. *a*, The usual site of the incision which, however, may be made at the midline or to the left of the midline. *b*, A withdrawn loop of transverse colon held up by means of a rubber catheter or a piece of umbilical tape. *c*, The approximation of adjoining limbs of intestine, which facilitates subsequent application of a clamp for crushing the spur. *d*, A transverse incision rather than a vertical incision averts the necessity of the additional incisions shown, through which the cut ends of the bowel are drawn as is indicated in *e*. Instead of making an independent incision the procedure may be done through part of the existing, or the extended principal, incision. *f*, Application of clamp for crushing the spur.

cases in which fecal fistulas develop from colonic wounds. The Devine type of colostomy (Fig. 28) is preferable because it everts spillage from the proximal to the distal loop, and because of the facility with which restitution of continuity of the intestinal lumen subsequently can be accomplished. The performance of *cecostomy* is, in general, of little value.

The conditions which require *resection of portions of the large intestine* are essentially identical with those which have been discussed in indicating the necessity for removal of segments of small intestine.

Drainage is important in the treatment of wounds of the large bowel, and it should be instituted when doubt as to the integrity of the suture line exists, as well as in every case of proved or questionable retroperitoneal injury.

Mortality Associated with Injuries of Large Intestine.—Uncomplicated perforations of the large intestine caused by a single, small missile, when associated with only slight spillage of semisolid fecal material, are attended by a relatively low mortality if early closure of the perforation is done. Large perforations, however, usually are followed by rapidly developing sepsis and many of the patients with such injuries die within a few hours. In the war of 1914–1918 the mortality record for wounds of the large intestine was 58.7 per cent, compared with a mortality of 65.9 per cent following wounds of the small intestine. The death rate following colonic injuries was greatly increased by the group of cases in which colostomy was performed, the mortality after suture of the colon being only slightly more than 50 per cent, while that following colostomy was 73.5 per cent. This does not mean that colostomy is necessarily a dangerous operation but that sepsis is likely to cause death in cases in which colostomy is required.

Wounds of Rectum

Injuries of the rectum are *comparatively infrequent;* they constituted only 2.4 per cent of the lesions of abdominal viscera in the war of 1914–1918. Lesions often associated are those of the bladder, the pelvic colon, and, less frequently, injuries of the small bowel.

Rectal lesions vary in size from small perforations, caused by minute projectiles or fragments of pelvic bone, to extensive lacerations. It is sometimes possible, by means of digital examination of the rectum, to detect a perforation or a spicule of bone which projects into the lumen; in other instances blood on the gloved examining finger may be the only indication of rectal injury. Eventually local tenderness, along with other evidences of infection of the perineum, indicate that there has been an extraperitoneal rectal wound.

The following aspects of rectal wounds must be considered: (1) The external damage may be very great, with tearing away of a large portion of the gluteal region. The anus and lower portion of the rectum may be completely avulsed or the lumen may be opened on one side only. If the projectile is small, the sphincter may be left intact. The injury may be limited to the portion of the rectum below the peritoneal reflection. In addition to peritonitis, infection in the perirectal extraperitoneal space is a frequent complication. Although even extensive wounds of the buttocks are not necessarily serious, there is danger of gas gangrene in the gluteal muscles. Wounds involving the sacrum without an opening in the bowel are frequently fatal because of infection of the presacral areolar tissue; however, pieces of shell protruding into the rectum on its posterolateral aspect have been removed and recovery has followed without any further surgical procedure. (2) The rectum may be wounded extraperitoneally, intraperitoneally, or both. Missiles which cause the injuries may take a side to side, anteroposterior or semi-vertical course. The side to side wounds are deceptive, their posterior situation suggesting that the missile has missed the bowel.

Treatment of Injuries of Rectum.—The treatment of rectal injuries associated with wounds of the buttock consists in excising all damaged tissue and, when possible, closing the rent in the bowel or sphincter, although sometimes it may be better to lay open the lower end of the canal by dividing the sphincter. If the peritoneum has been opened, the abdominal cavity should be closed off by sutures. The expediency of colostomy must in part be determined by the difficulty of otherwise keeping the patient clean and comfortable; usually it is necessary when the whole lower segment of the bowel has been carried away. In such cases, the lumen can be closed by sutures or a purse-string ligature, either of which help to limit contamination of the pelvis while adhesions are forming. If colostomy is necessary, transverse colostomy is best because of the ease of cleaning the opening, of fitting a colostomy bag, or of subsequent closure.

When a projectile has traversed the pelvis, exploratory celiotomy should be done. If the peritoneal surface has escaped, the abdomen can be closed and the rectal wound exposed exteriorly. Anterior wounds usually can be sutured easily, except when they are deep in the pelvis. The bottom of the rectovesical pouch can be shut off by suturing the peritoneum over it.

Mortality Associated with Wounds of Rectum.—The mortality

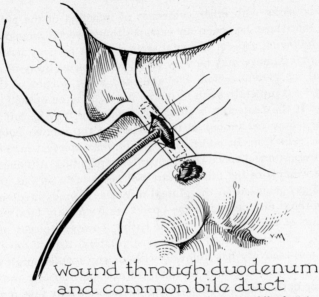

Wound through duodenum
and common bile duct

Fig. 29.—Introduction of a T tube into the common bile duct to divert bile
when the retroduodenal portion of the bile duct has been injured. Casualties to
whom such a procedure can be applied are rarely encountered, and usually they
die because of the almost invariably associated duodenal, pancreatic, or other
injuries.

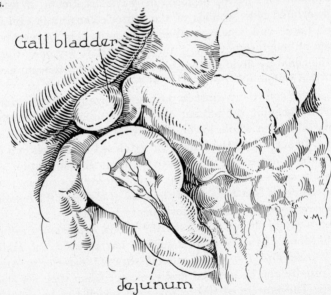

Fig. 30.—The sites of incision for performance of cholecystojejunostomy.
This procedure, as well as such less desirable ones as cholecystogastrostomy and
cholecystoduodenostomy, can be employed in cases of injury of the common bile
duct.

following wounds of the rectum in the war of 1914–1918 was 45.19 per cent. Death is usually due to rapidly advancing sepsis in the retroperitoneal tissues, or to spreading peritonitis.

Injuries of Gallbladder and Bile Ducts

The seriousness of injuries to the gallbladder and extrahepatic bile passages is frequently increased by associated wounds of the duodenum, the pancreas, or the pancreatic ducts. Obscuring hematomas usually interfere with identification and repair of injuries of the bile ducts; these structures may be damaged beyond repair. Short circuiting operations, such as cholecystoduodenostomy, cholecysto-gastrostomy, or cholecystojejunostomy are feasible only under exceptional circumstances. Simple injuries of the gallbladder can be treated by cholecystostomy, cholecystectomy or, rarely, by suture of the wound (Figs. 29, 30).

INJURIES OF MESENTERY

Wounds of the mesentery may be of all sorts, varying from simple perforations to irregular tears. They may occur without a lesion of the

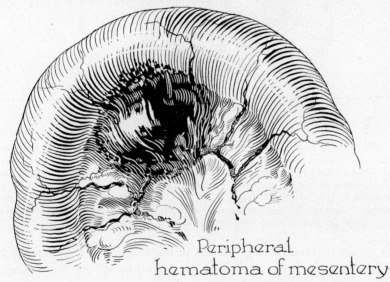

Peripheral hematoma of mesentery

Fig. 31.—Hematoma near the junction of the mesentery with the intestine. Hematomas in this location which extend beneath the serous coat of the bowel should be incised, for they may obscure intestinal perforations. The injury to terminal blood vessels responsible for the formation of hematomas in this position occasionally causes such a degree of ischemia of a small segment of adjoining bowel as to necessitate intestinal resection.

bowel. Large segments of intestine sometimes are torn away from the mesentery, with resulting massive hemorrhage but without associated perforations of the intestine.

Injury to the mesenteric blood vessels may be followed by hemorrhage into the peritoneal cavity, between the leaves of the mesentery, or into the retroperitoneal space. Bleeding into any of these regions is usually greater if the wound is located in the central zone or near the

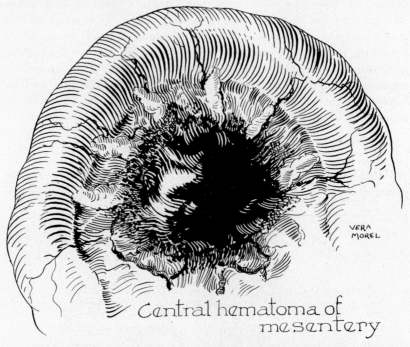

Central hematoma of mesentery

Fig. 32.—Hematoma located in the central zone of the mesentery. Because of the opportunities for collateral circulation in this region, small hematomas here are not likely to be associated with serious impairment of the blood supply to the nearby intestine, and they usually should be left alone. However, if a hematoma in this position is large, if it can be seen to be enlarging, or if there is active bleeding through an opening in it, it should be opened widely and search made for the point of unarrested bleeding.

base of the mesentery. The amount of detachment of the mesentery which may occur without consequent devitalization of the attached intestine varies greatly. Although separation for as short a distance as $\frac{3}{4}$ inch (about 2 cm.) can so interfere with the blood supply to the intestine as to make resection advisable, in other instances a much greater amount of separation may exist without causing serious ischemia of the bowel. The presence of a hematoma between the leaves of the mesentery makes it difficult to locate the ends of the torn vessels and to determine whether or not spontaneous hemostasis has occurred. Also, injury to the intestine at its junction with the mesentery is often obscured by a hematoma between the leaves of the

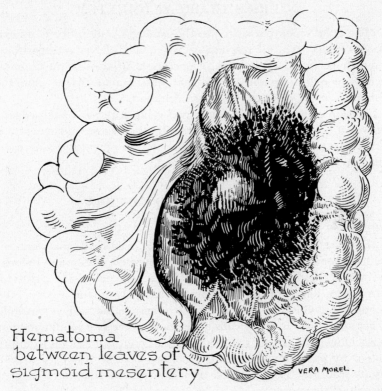

Fig. 33.—Hematoma located between the leaves of the mesentery of the sigmoid. Hematomas resulting from injuries to the large branches of the superior or inferior mesenteric arteries, near the root of the mesentery, sometimes extend far in the retroperitoneal space, even reaching into the pelvis. Under such circumstances, location of the point of bleeding is difficult or impossible and, because of the danger of exposing the retroperitoneal space to infection, and because of the possibility of causing more injury to blood vessels, search for the torn vessel usually should be made only when it is believed, or known, that a damaged vessel is still bleeding.

mesentery, or by one extending beneath the serosal layer of the intestine (Figs. 31, 32, 33).

Repair of injuries to the mesentery is usually best accomplished by grasping the torn or cut edges with forceps and ligating the tissue within their grasp. Approximation of the mesentery by suturing is likely to result in free bleeding or formation of a hematoma between the leaves of the mesentery, due to perforation of an obscured blood vessel. Mesenteric injury may necessitate intestinal resection, even though the corresponding segment of bowel has not been directly damaged.

INJURIES TO GREAT OMENTUM

The great omentum is frequently damaged, and injury to omental *blood vessels* is often responsible for much of the intraperitoneal hemorrhage found at the time of operation. Injuries of the omentum include punctate wounds, tears and detachment of the omentum. Hematomas between its layers are common.

Ligation of the bleeding points and tying together of the edges of rents is a satisfactory method of treating the less serious omental injuries. More or less complete resection of the omentum is necessary when it has been extensively damaged.

WOUNDS OF SOLID VISCERA

Wounds of Liver

Because of its large size the liver is *often injured,* and wounds of the liver comprised 13.3 per cent of all traumatic abdominal lesions in the war of 1914–1918. Approximately 75 per cent of the hepatic injuries were uncomplicated. Associated wounds, in the order of their frequency, involve the colon, stomach, and kidneys. The possibility of hepatic injury must be considered in the presence of all abdomino-thoracic wounds on the right side of the body. In addition to injuries caused by penetrating projectiles, serious hepatic trauma frequently results from fractured ribs and from blunt force. Blast injuries of the liver may also occur.

Depending on the cause of the injury, various types of hepatic lesions are: (1) the cleancut wound, which may be caused by a projectile, an indriven rib, or by a bayonet or knife; (2) perforations or punctate injuries; (3) furrowing wounds; (4) splits or radiating fissures; (5) crateriform wounds; (6) ragged wounds; (7) coexisting wounds of different types (Fig. 34).

Because of the fixation and friability of the liver, hepatic wounds are often of a stellate or fracture type. The liver may be extensively ruptured by relatively small missiles, and injuries due to falls, or blows by blunt objects, may cause fragmentation of this organ. Practically the entire liver may be shattered, and considerable portions of it may be torn loose, especially from the anterior edge, and may either lie free in the abdomen or be carried completely away from the body.

The torn surface of the liver, after twelve to twenty-four hours, becomes a dirty yellowish brown; later it may be a vivid yellow due to staining with bile.

Symptoms of Hepatic Injury.—*Hemorrhage* always follows injuries of the liver and varies from slight oozing to rapidly fatal loss of

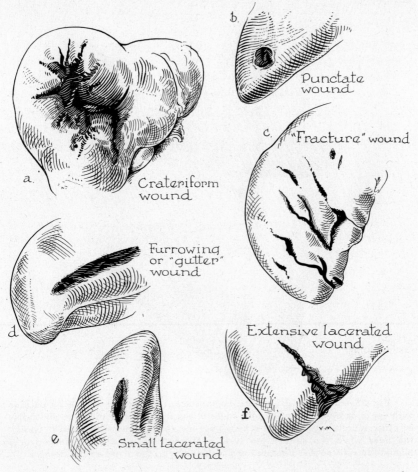

Fig. 34.—Various types of wounds of the liver. Except for punctate wounds, indicated in *b*, and furrowing or gutter wounds, indicated in *d*, the injuries illustrated may be caused by blunt force as well as by projectiles or indriven objects.

blood. Symptoms of *peritoneal irritation* result from blood and sometimes bile in the peritoneal cavity. When patients are seen two to three days after the injury, there is frequently slight *jaundice*.

Secondary Hemorrhage from Liver.—Secondary hemorrhage from

the liver can occur several days following injury and is commonly
accompanied by *pain, distention* of the abdomen, rise of *temperature,*
and *acceleration* of the pulse, associated with *pallor, restlessness,* and
rapid *loss of strength.* With these general symptoms, a localized swelling which may be indistinguishable from a secondary abscess usually
develops.

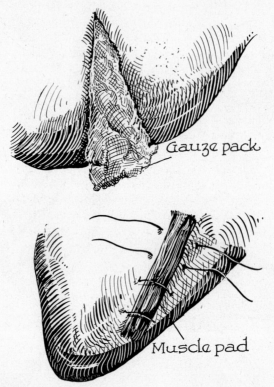

Fig. 35.—Methods of arresting hemorrhage from hepatic wounds by packing
with gauze or by suturing the torn edges of the liver. A strip of rectus abdominis
or other muscle serves as a resilient pad and reduces the likelihood of tearing
the liver when the sutures are tied. If the muscle is partially macerated, a
hemostatic substance is liberated and contributes to the arrest of bleeding.

Treatment of Injuries of Liver.—If they occur alone, hepatic
injuries are frequently best treated conservatively. In the presence of
small wounds, *spontaneous hemostasis* is usually as effective as that
which could be accomplished by any surgical procedure. The increased respiratory movements incident to anesthesia, along with
dislodgment of blood clots and separations of the liver from the diaphragm or the abdominal wall when the abdomen is opened, some-

times result in renewal of hepatic bleeding. If hepatic injury is very extensive, and especially when there has been loss of hepatic tissue, little can be accomplished by operation. Between these extremes, however, are the still actively bleeding wounds, which can be *sutured* or *packed* (Fig. 35). (See also Figs. 12, 14, 43.)

For exposure and treatment of hepatic wounds a *right subcostal* incision is best; sometimes this should be supplemented by division or resection of costal cartilages to facilitate exposure of the dome of the liver. On the other hand, a *median* or *paramedian* approach often affords adequate exposure and may better permit location and repair of injuries in other parts of the abdomen. If the projectile has entered through the thorax and lodged in the liver, a *transpleural* approach may be best.

If a small wound of the liver is found it should be left alone if there is no active hemorrhage. When possible, control of bleeding from the liver should be accomplished by *suturing* instead of depending on packs. In placing sutures in the liver, the needle should enter at some distance from the lacerated edge and the suture, introduced in mattress fashion, should be tied loosely enough to avoid tearing. When it is impossible to control bleeding from the liver except by packing with gauze, *plain dry gauze* is better than iodoform gauze, as use of the latter may be followed by serious toxic effects due to absorption of iodoform. When the hepatic wound is small, hemostasis may be facilitated by applying or suturing a piece of *macerated muscle* to the bleeding surface of the liver. Bleeding from a torn hepatic surface sometimes can be rapidly arrested by topical application of a preparation of *thrombin. Temporary control of bleeding from the liver* may be accomplished by *compression* of the *hepatic artery* and *portal vein* where they course in the edge of the *gastrohepatic omentum,* as shown in Fig. 14.

Hepatic tissue which has been detached should be removed, not only to avert the development of autolytic peritonitis, but to reduce the danger of peritoneal infection with anaerobic micro-organisms.

Although outpouring of *bile* from lacerated surfaces of the liver usually is not detectable at the time of operation, it may occur subsequently and produce *chemical peritonitis.* Accumulation of bile in the region of the liver or in the pelvis may require drainage. If oozing of bile due to severance of large bile passages is observed at operation, the introduction of drains may obviate biliary peritonitis.

An hepatic *abscess* may develop around a retained projectile and can prove fatal unless adequate drainage is provided. If possible, the foreign body should be removed.

Mortality Associated with Hepatic Wounds.—The mortality rate associated with wounds of the liver was 66.27 per cent in the war of 1914–1918. Injuries to the intrahepatic bile passages did not seem to increase the gravity of hepatic injuries to any appreciable extent.

Wounds of Spleen

Wounds of the spleen occur less frequently than those of the liver; only forty-nine wounds of the spleen were recorded as being observed in the American Expeditionary Force in the war of 1914–1918. Many of the patients with splenic wounds had complicating lesions, which usually involved the *kidneys, stomach,* and *colon.*

Splenic injury must always be considered in cases in which the left side of the chest or abdomen has sustained severe trauma, whether due to blunt force or to a penetrating object, and the possibility of perforation of the spleen by a fractured rib should be borne in mind (Fig. 36).

Splenic wounds may be of all types, including perforations, tears, splits in the capsule, avulsion of poles, hemisection, division of the pedicle, total detachment, or almost complete disruption. Formation of a subcapsular hematoma sometimes follows splenic trauma and, either spontaneously or after secondary trauma, the hematoma may rupture and cause serious delayed hemorrhage even weeks or months later.

When injuries of the spleen are located near the large splenic blood vessels, massive intra-abdominal hemorrhage almost invariably occurs. However, small punctate wounds of the spleen, if located near the poles or the convex surface are often not followed by continued hemorrhage. The splenic pulp has been found bleeding forty-eight hours after injury but hemorrhage usually ceases after ten hours.

Symptoms of Splenic Injury.—The symptoms resulting from injury of the spleen are principally those of *shock* and *hemorrhage,* along with signs of *peritoneal irritation* caused by blood in the peritoneal cavity. If bleeding from the spleen is slight, determinations of specific gravity of the blood and of mean corpuscular volume may be required to reveal the existence and continuance of bleeding. When injuries of the spleen are due to penetrating wounds, there may be oozing of blood from the wound in the abdominal wall. Although blood may accumulate in the left flank following splenic injury, damming up of the blood in the left loin is not frequently detectable.

Treatment of Splenic Injuries.—A *transverse* or *subcostal* incision affords optimal exposure of the spleen but the presence of other abdominal injuries may require a *paramedian* incision. The latter type of incision may be extended transversely if necessary.

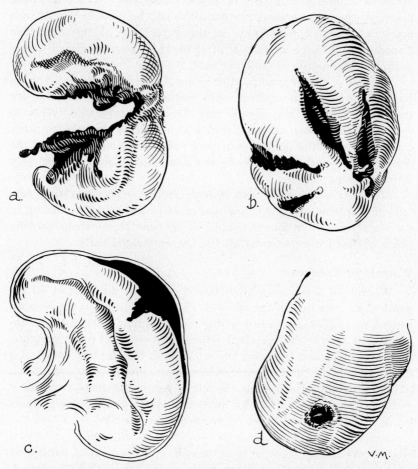

Fig. 36.—Several types of injury of the spleen. Splenectomy is the only satisfactory procedure when lesions such as those shown in *a* and *b* are found, and, because of the danger of secondary hemorrhage, the spleen usually should be removed when a subcapsular hematoma, indicated in *c*, is present, even though there is no bleeding at the time of operation. Except for the type of wound shown in *d*, the lesions represented can be produced by blunt force as well as by projectiles or other indriven objects. When a small, punctate wound is located near one of the poles, as in *d* and there is no bleeding at the time of operation, it may be best not to perform splenectomy if there are many injuries to other organs, or if the patient is suffering from shock and hemorrhage.

Suture of the spleen is not as satisfactory as is suture of the liver and, if there are extensive lacerations of the spleen, *splenectomy* is to be preferred because of the possible continuation of bleeding following suture. If only a punctate injury of the spleen exists, and especially if this is located near a pole or at a considerable distance from the hilum, neither splenectomy nor suture should be done unless there is active bleeding. Splenectomy, in the experience of the American Expeditionary Force in the war of 1914–1918, was associated with a mortality of practically 100 per cent.

Because of the frequency, after splenectomy, of *progressive thrombosis* beginning in the splenic vein, postoperative heparinization for the prevention of this complication has been suggested. When a wound of the spleen is associated with extensive damage to other organs, or when the patient is in very poor condition, packing of the splenic wound with gauze may be expedient, but is never a thoroughly satisfactory procedure.

Mortality Associated with Splenic Injury.—The mortality rate following splenic wounds in the war of 1914–1918 was, according to various reports, from 50 per cent to 63 per cent. Hemorrhage was the cause of death in practically all the uncomplicated cases.

Wounds of Pancreas

Wounds of the pancreas comprised about 0.2 per cent of all abdominal injuries in the war of 1914–1918. In addition to the wounds caused by projectiles, injury of the pancreas may be due to its impingement against the vertebral column as a result of blunt pressure, such as that caused by being thrown against the steering wheel of a motor vehicle. In cases of pancreatic trauma, the frequent association of injuries to the great vessels, the bile or pancreatic ducts, or the duodenum, is responsible either for immediate death or for many patients being in hopeless condition on reaching the hospital.

Symptoms of Pancreatic Injury.—Pancreatic injuries do not cause characteristic early signs or symptoms. Even at operation, pancreatic wounds are often overlooked, especially when obscured by a retroperitoneal hematoma. The first evidence of injury to the pancreas may be that produced by the development, weeks after the injury was sustained, of a pseudocyst. Elevated values for blood sugar, as well as for blood lipase and diastase, may follow pancreatic injury.

Treatment of Injury to Pancreas.—Especially when the injury is in the region of the head of the pancreas there is little possibility of successful surgical treatment because of the frequently associated extensive injuries to the bile or pancreatic ducts, or to the duodenum. About all that can be done in most cases is to establish drainage, including cholecystojejunostomy, or to institute drainage by introducing a T tube into the common bile duct. In rare instances, when the lesion is located in the tail of the pancreas, it may be possible to resect the portion which lies to the left of the site of injury, and to close over the cut end. If injuries involve the head of the pancreas, the possibility of performing resection, such as may be done for car-

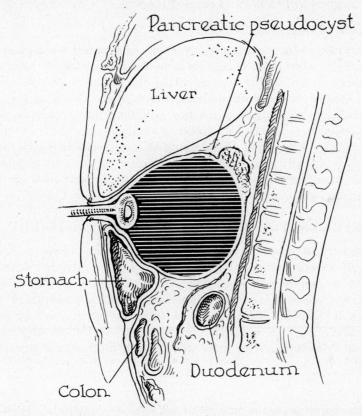

Fig. 37.—Method of marsupializing a traumatic pseudocyst of the pancreas. Depending on the position and size of the cyst, it can be approached through the gastrohepatic ligament, the gastrocolic ligament or, rarely, through the transverse mesocolon.

cinoma of the head of the pancreas, may be considered but this is not likely to be feasible.

Marsupialization of a traumatic pseudocyst (Fig. 37) of the pancreas is usually a satisfactory method of treatment. However, complete excision of the pseudocyst has been advocated because pancreatic fistulas have been observed in some cases in which marsupialization was done. Late operation also may be necessary for drainage of a pancreatic abscess, or for removal of a foreign body lodged within the gland.

Prognosis and Mortality Associated with Injury of Pancreas.— The prognosis is extremely *poor* in cases of pancreatic injury. The mortality is *almost 100 per cent,* even among those patients who survive long enough to reach a general hospital.

Wounds of Suprarenal Glands

Because of their small size, the suprarenal glands are *seldom injured.* Even when those glands are wounded, recognition of the injury is difficult or impossible because of the absence of distinctive symptoms, because of the position and smallness of the glands, or because of obscuring hematomas. An entire suprarenal gland may be torn away, and damage to the corresponding kidney is associated with most such injuries. The extent of the injury or the interference with blood supply practically always *precludes surgical repair,* and treatment either is entirely conservative, or consists of extirpation of the damaged gland, usually along with the corresponding kidney.

EVISCERATION FOLLOWING ABDOMINAL INJURY

Abdominal viscera, including the omentum, often protrude through wounds in the parietal wall. Wounds of the extruded parts are sometimes present and, when the opening through which eventration has taken place is small, strangulation caused by constriction and edema at the point of emergence adds to the damage resulting from trauma, chilling and contamination. Evisceration of upper abdominal viscera is accompanied by more shock than is protrusion of the small bowel.

Omentum

The omentum is the structure most frequently extruded. It either is carried out by the projectile or, more commonly, is forced out through the wound of entrance or exit by intra-abdominal pressure. Depending on the site of injury, protrusion may even take place through the costal interspaces or between fragments of fractured ribs. In abdominothoracic wounds the omentum may plug the rent in the diaphragm. Strangulation of the omentum between the layers of the abdominal wall may occur.

When the omentum has remained outside of the abdomen for some time, and especially when it has been strangulated, edema may make its replacement impossible unless the opening through which protrusion occurred is enlarged or a part of the extruded portion is resected. It is usually advisable to withdraw additional omentum, so that resection can be performed through a clean and undamaged portion. Before operative treatment was customary in the management of abdominal injuries, omental tags frequently were allowed to slough off and this is still probably the best course if the patient is seen late after injury.

Stomach

The stomach may be herniated alone or in conjunction with the transverse colon, the omentum, the small intestine or the spleen.

Liver

Although this organ is sometimes partly herniated, its size and fixation make extensive protrusion of the liver impossible. Injuries of sufficient size to permit protrusion of the liver are almost invariably fatal, due to severe hemorrhage.

Small Intestine

Because of its extent, size and mobility, the small intestine is, next to the omentum, the most commonly eviscerated abdominal organ. Wounds in extruded loops of the small bowel are not uncommon. Strangulation sometimes follows when protrusion occurs through a small parietal wound.

Colon

The transverse colon is likely to be herniated along with the omentum and sometimes with the stomach and the small intestine.

INJURIES TO MAJOR BLOOD VESSELS

Injuries to large blood vessels of the abdomen usually result in *death from hemorrhage* before the patients reach a surgical unit. Bleeding from the *inferior vena cava* has been controlled successfully by suture, or by one or more forceps applied to the rent in the vein and left in position for some days, with the handles projecting. *Vascular suture,* with reinforcement of the site of repair by a muscle flap, a piece of fascia or a tab of fat, is at times possible. When the extent of injury to the iliac arteries makes their *ligation* imperative, a single injection of 95 per cent alcohol, or repeated injections of 1 per cent solution of procaine, in the region of the appropriate lumbar sympathetic ganglia, may avert gangrene of the parts distal to the site of ligation (Fig. 38).

When an aneurysm follows injury of an iliac vessel, *endo-*

aneurysmorrhaphy or *ligation* may be necessary, after preliminary interruption of conduction through the lumbar sympathetic nerves.

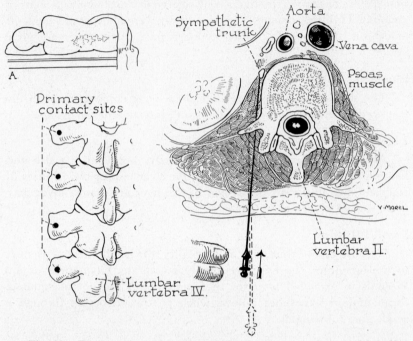

Fig. 38.—Position of patient, anatomic landmarks, and method of injecting in the region of the lumbar sympathetic ganglia, to prevent ischemia of the lower extremities when it is necessary to ligate the aorta or the common or external iliac arteries. The sites of puncture are two fingerbreadths lateral to the midline. After primary contact has been made with the respective transverse processes, the needles are slightly withdrawn, redirected so as to pass by the transverse processes, and then introduced two fingerbreadths deeper than when primary contact was made.

WOUNDS OF GENITO-URINARY ORGANS

Injuries to genito-urinary organs are frequently encountered in the course of operations for other wounds of the abdominal region, and incisions sometimes must be modified to permit exploration or repair of such wounds. In the instance of nurses or other female casualties, incisions which will permit access to the uterus and its adnexae may be necessary.

Wounds of Kidneys

Injuries of these organs constituted 6.3 per cent of all abdominal injuries in the war of 1914–1918, and in half of the cases there were no complications.

About a third of all wounds of the right kidney are complicated by injury to the *liver,* and wounds of the left kidney are almost as often accompanied by *splenic* lesions. Hollow viscera most often wounded in conjunction with the kidneys are the *small bowel* or the *colon.* Wounds of the renal blood vessels are often fatal because of severe hemorrhage, and injuries to the renal arteries or their branches

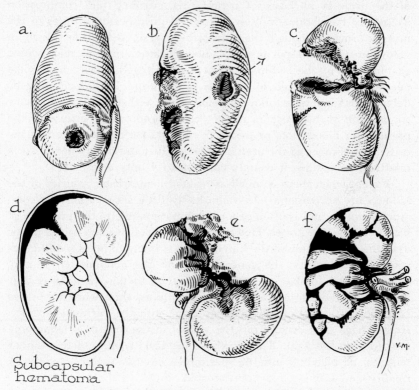

Fig. 39.—Various types of renal injuries, *a, b, c, d, e, f.* The injury shown in *d* is associated with a subcapsular hematoma. For the smaller wounds, entirely conservative methods or suture yield the best results. Even when the extensive character of a renal wound requires that nephrectomy be performed, it is often advisable to delay this procedure for several days, or at least until the patient has recovered from shock.

may be followed by extensive infarction. Injuries limited to the renal pelvis are comparatively rare. Wounds of the kidney may be of any type from a simple perforating wound to extensive laceration or disruption of the organ. Other injuries, such as scores, furrows, tears in the capsule, avulsion of the poles, and hemisection, will also be seen. The kidney may be found lying loose, while at other times the blood vessels are completely divided, with the ureter remaining intact. Recognition of renal injury is often difficult because of the presence of a perirenal hematoma (Fig. 39).

Diagnosis of Renal Injury.—*Hematuria* is present in about 90 per cent of cases. It is usually detectable immediately after injury, and is as a rule proportionate to the extent of renal damage. Examination of the urine in all cases of penetrating, crushing, and compression wounds of the abdomen often will reveal unsuspected injuries of the urinary tract. Although there may be grossly detectable blood in voided urine or in a specimen obtained by catheterization, microscopic examination of the sediment from a centrifuged specimen may be necessary to reveal red blood cells in the urine. Hematuria may be delayed for some time following renal injury, either because of urinary suppression such as occurs in the "crush syndrome," because of the presence of blood clots or pieces of renal tissue in the ureter, or because of severance of the ureter. Although hematuria may persist for a relatively long time, it usually continues for only a few days.

Except when there is much associated hemorrhage, injuries of the kidneys are accompanied by remarkably *little shock. Pain* is a common symptom and is often of a colicky nature, due to the presence of blood clots in the ureter. However, if there is distention of the pelvis or of the true capsule of the kidney, pain is likely to be of a dull character. The pain may be generalized over the abdomen or it may extend to the lumbar or sacral regions, or to the shoulder or hip. *Nausea* and *vomiting* are frequent symptoms, even when there has been no extravasation of blood or urine into the peritoneal cavity. *Hemorrhage* may occur from the wound in the loin, or a hematoma may form in the flank. There may be localized *rigidity* of the lumbar muscles, or bleeding into the peritoneal cavity, so that *tenderness, rigidity* and *dulness,* may be detected.

Secondary hemorrhage is a fairly frequent, and sometimes fatal, late complication. It occurs most often during the second or third week after injury, and usually when the urine is contaminated. Delayed hemorrhage may start without there having been primary hemorrhage. Unlike primary hemorrhage, recurrent bleeding is often accompanied by clotting of the blood in the bladder.

External leakage of urine may occur when the pelvis of the kidney has been opened, or when the ureter has been torn, but is seldom present when the injury involves only the renal parenchyma.

Roentgenologic examination may demonstrate absence of the outline of a psoas muscle, flexion of the spinal column toward the affected side, or change in the size and contour of the renal outline. Intravenous or retrograde pyelography may further reveal the character and extent of a renal injury, and anterior displacement of a ureter as revealed by a lateral pyelogram is evidence of a perinephritic accumulation of pus, blood or urine.

Treatment of Renal Injuries.—Entirely *conservative* treatment of wounds of the kidneys is usually advisable in the instance of closed injuries caused by blunt force, but *suture* of the kidney or *nephrectomy* may be necessary. Massive hemorrhage, urinary leakage, advancing symptoms of sepsis, or the presence of a large retained foreign body, are the principal indications for operation.

When renal injury is suspected in a case in which operation is required for other abdominal injuries, the incision should if possible be made *transversely* or *obliquely,* at a level which will facilitate exposure and treatment of the possible renal wounds.

When there is *no active bleeding* at the time of operation, it is usually best to do nothing, or only to provide external drainage. As in hepatic injuries, hemorrhage from the kidney often recurs following removal of blood clots in the region of the wound.

Renal injuries, discovered in the course of an operation through a *paramedian* incision, often must be treated by merely introducing rubber tissue drains or gauze into the region of the injury and allowing the drains or gauze to make their exit through the usually existing wound in the loin. The torn peritoneum in the region of the wound should, if possible, be sutured to prevent passage of urine into the peritoneal cavity. Obscuring perirenal hematomas frequently hamper treatment and, in some instances, provision of drainage is all that can be done. When a small missile is found, it often can be removed through the existing incision in the anterior abdominal wall. It may even be possible, through such an incision, to trim away devitalized renal tissue.

Treatment of *extensive* renal wounds which occur in conjunction with multiple intraperitoneal visceral injuries is usually unsatisfactory and compromise methods are often necessary. A shattered pole, or hemisection, of a kidney may be found which, if existing alone, would warrant nephrectomy; but the patient's general condition and the necessity of repairing numerous other injuries may make it seem unwise to remove the kidney, either through an extension of the existing incision or through a separate incision in the loin.

If a patient's condition does not permit nephrectomy, and if bleeding cannot be controlled by packing, it may be necessary to place clamps on the renal blood vessels, leaving the clamps in place, with their handles protruding through the wound in the abdominal wall.

Especially when renal injury is uncomplicated, bleeding may be controlled by placing interlacing ribbon catgut around the kidney and beneath its capsule.

Incision and drainage of a *perinephritic abscess* or evacuation of *extravasated urine and blood* through an incision in the loin may be necessary as a secondary operation. It also may be necessary in cases in which prior treatment has been by entirely conservative methods.

Mortality Associated with Renal Injury.—The mortality attending uncomplicated renal injury varies from 25 to 30 per cent. Early death is usually due to hemorrhage, whereas sepsis and secondary hemorrhage are the chief causes of late death.

Wounds of Ureters

Wounds of the ureters are rare, but preoperative recognition of the possibility of such injuries is important because introduction of a ureteral catheter, before the abdomen has been opened, facilitates their discovery and repair.

When wounds of the ureter are *small,* they can sometimes be satisfactorily sutured. If the wound is near the bladder, the ureter may be implanted in the bladder. If the wound is *large,* or if there has been so much loss of substance that repair or anastomosis is impossible, it may be feasible only to introduce a drain for the external conduction of urine, or to perform nephrostomy, but if possible the ureter should be sufficiently mobilized to permit bringing the sectioned end to the surface of the skin where its wall is sutured to the surrounding edge of skin. To avert formation of a *calculus* or a *stricture,* care must be taken to avoid introduction of suture material into the lumen of the ureter. Fistulas resulting from wounds of the ureter often close spontaneously. Even though nephrectomy may eventually be necessary because of a persistent urinary fistula, *primary nephrectomy usually is not advisable.*

Wounds of Bladder

Wounds of the bladder comprised approximately 5 per cent of all abdominal lesions in the war of 1914–1918. The majority of vesical wounds were complicated by injuries to the intestine or bony pelvis. Wounds of the rectum were found in from 10 to 15 per cent of the cases but injury of the prostate gland was comparatively rare. The small intestine is the organ most frequently wounded in conjunction with the bladder. The wound of entrance is most frequently situated posteriorly and there is often no wound of exit.

Lesions of the bladder may be extraperitoneal or intraperitoneal, and they vary considerably both in size and character. Perforation of the bladder may be caused either by a projectile or by a spicule of pelvic bone. The "explosive" type of wound, whether due to blunt force or a projectile, usually occurs when the bladder is full (Fig. 40).

Symptoms, Diagnosis, and Complications of Vesical Wounds.—Hematuria may follow either penetrating or nonpenetrating vesical wounds. *Micturition is sometimes impossible. Discharge of urine*

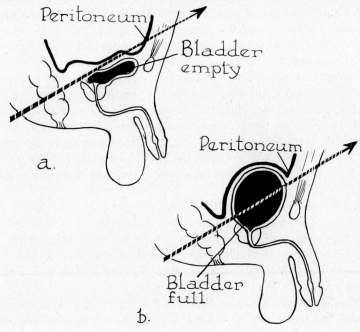

Fig. 40.—Depending on whether the bladder is empty or filled, it may escape injury or be damaged by a missile traversing a given course. When a projectile strikes a distended bladder, an "explosive" type of injury may be produced as a result of the incompressibility of the fluid contents.

through the parietal wound of entry or exit is uncommon if the wound is small.

Hemorrhage from wounds of the bladder is usually not serious. Bleeding into the bladder suggests an extraperitoneal lesion and, with this type of injury there may be an obvious swelling above the inguinal ligament due to a large hematoma in the vicinity of the visceral wound. An empty bladder, especially when associated with signs of peritoneal irritation, suggests the existence of intraperitoneal perforation, with leakage of urine into the peritoneal cavity.

Pelvic cellulitis is likely to follow extraperitoneal vesical wounds and, in cases of long standing, necrosis of bone, formation of calculi, and persistent cystitis are frequent complications.

Treatment of Vesical Wounds.—Access to the sites of *intraperitoneal wounds* is usually best gained through a midline, subumbilical incision extending down to the symphysis pubis. Intraperitoneal wounds are as a rule easily sutured, except when situated at the bottom of the rectovesical pouch. Before closing an intraperitoneal wound, examination should be made for other wounds or for a foreign body. Suprapubic cystostomy, performed either through a part of the original wound or through a new opening in the bladder, is usually necessary to provide constant drainage of the bladder following repair of vesical wounds.

Extraperitoneal injuries are best treated by wide incisions down to the vesical wounds followed by suture if possible. Complete drainage of the soft tissues, including the prevesical space, must then be provided. Drainage of the bladder should be provided for by means of suprapubic cystostomy. In some instances the original wound can be used for introduction of the catheter. If the wound in the bladder cannot be sutured, a drain extending down to the wound should be introduced.

An obscuring perivesical hematoma often makes the location of vesical injuries difficult, and when there is uncertainty as to their existence, suprapubic cystostomy should be done and drainage of the extravesical space provided. When the wound is located on the rectal surface of the bladder, it is necessary to close the wound by the transvesical route.

Mortality and Causes of Death Following Vesical Wounds.—The average mortality rate following uncomplicated vesical wounds is about 50 per cent. When the vesical injury is associated with a lesion of the small intestine, the mortality rate may be as high as 75 or 80 per cent. The causes of death are *sepsis, peritonitis* or, more rarely, secondary *hemorrhage* from the pelvic vessels.

Wounds of Genito-urinary Organs Distal to Bladder

Injuries to the vasa deferentia and spermatic cords are almost invariably obscured by hematomas and, even if recognized, are usually irreparable. When the prostate gland or posterior urethra is injured, suprapubic cystostomy is usually the best procedure, although perineal urethrostomy is sometimes preferable. If the urethra has been completely divided, at least partial approximation of the severed ends should be done, if circumstances permit.

Prophylaxis against Infection in Cases of Injury of Urogenital Tract

In anticipation of infection after injuries to the various parts of the urogenital tract, urinary antiseptic substances such as derivatives of *mandelic acid* or drugs of the *sulfonamide* group should be given as soon as possible.

ABDOMINOTHORACIC INJURIES

These complicated wounds comprised 4.6 per cent of the thoracic injuries brought to the evacuation hospitals of the American Expeditionary Force in the war of 1914–1918; other statistics based on experiences in that war show that in about 12 per cent of all wounds both the abdominal and thoracic cavities were involved. If only cases in which operation was performed are taken into account, the ratio is still about 12 per cent. These wounds are most often confined to one side, although the side of the chest opposite to that of the abdominal wound may be involved. Wounds low enough to involve both sides of the diaphragm are usually immediately fatal. Both sides are equally often affected and the mortality is the same whichever side is injured. In approximately a third of the cases a hollow abdominal organ is penetrated, and complicating wounds of the liver are more common than are those of the spleen.

Symptoms of Abdominothoracic Injuries

The characteristic manifestations of abdominothoracic wounds are sudden *pain* in the abdomen at the time of the receipt of the wound; *dyspnea; hemothorax;* abdominal *rigidity* over the corresponding half of the abdomen, especially in its upper part; and *shock,* which is dependent partially on the degree of hemorrhage and partially on the respiratory distress. *Vomiting* may occur and there may also be localized *tenderness.* The development of tension *pneumothorax* in cases in which there are relatively small thoracic wounds may cause even more serious respiratory and circulatory difficulty than is ordinarily present when "blowing" or "sucking" wounds exist.

Treatment of Abdominothoracic Injuries

The chief indications for *immediate treatment* of the thoracic element of these wounds are the presence of: (1) an open "blowing" or "sucking" wound, (2) a "stove in" or unstable chest wall, (3) retention in the thorax of a large missile, (4) tension pneumothorax.

The following *general principles* for the management of patients with abdominothoracic wounds have been established:

1. When there is a through-and-through abdominothoracic wound on the right side inflicted by only a small fragment, or if a fragment is retained in an inaccessible part of the liver, active surgical treatment may not be required unless there is evidence of continuing hemorrhage.

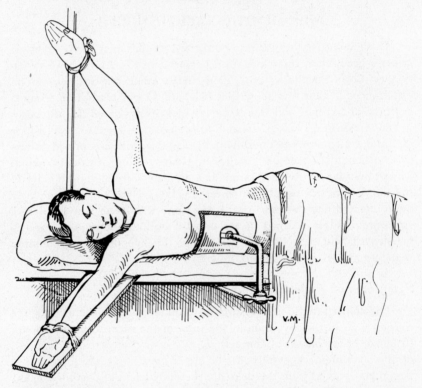

Fig. 41.—Position of patient and methods of fixation and support which facilitate exposure and operative procedures in cases of abdominothoracic trauma. The left wrist is fastened to an infusion stand, and the right arm is extended on a board to permit administration of an infusion or a transfusion.

2. When there is a small wound in the thorax and evidence of abdominal injury demanding operation, the abdominal lesion should be given priority, and operation should be done through an appropriately placed abdominal incision. The thorax may require no special attention.

3. When there is extensive through-and-through injury of the thorax, or if severe injury has been caused by a missile of

moderate size which is retained, the thoracic injury should be dealt with first, the abdomen sometimes being approached through the diaphragm.

If the thoracic wound is a *"blowing"* one, it should be closed by suture in which muscular layers are included. No "blowing" thoracic wound should be allowed to pass even the first aid station without closure. If tension pneumothorax follows a valvular thoracic injury, the air in the pleural cavity should be removed by aspiration and a piece of rubber tissue or vaseline gauze should be placed over the wound to prevent further ingress of air. If the chest wall is unstable, tight dressings should be applied to prevent paradoxical movement. The position and support of the patient on the operating table as represented in Fig. 41 is one which is often satisfactory for the definitive treatment of abdominothoracic wounds.

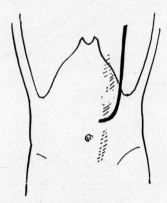

Fig. 42.—"Hockey-stick" incision, which is useful in some cases of abdomino-thoracic wounds.

A wound on the *left side, above* the level of the *eighth rib,* with associated *high abdominal* injury, can best be exposed by a vertical incision beginning on the thoracic wall near the thoracic wound. The ribs are sectioned in order to allow access to the thorax, and a prolongation of the wound downward opens the abdomen; at times, this lower extension can be continued obliquely forward (Fig. 42). An alternate method is to make a transpleural approach to the upper part of the abdomen, using an incision which is roughly transverse. A rib can be resected, or access can be had through an intercostal space with the aid of rib spreaders. The thoracic wound is dissected and any soiled parts of ribs, or loose fragments of bone are removed. With fresh instruments the pleural cavity is explored and any lesions en-

countered are treated. The wound in the diaphragm is then sought and
enlarged up to 5 or 6 inches (about 13 to 15 cm.); this exposure gives
a satisfactory approach to the abdomen. It is generally wise to obliterate the lowest part of the pleural space by suturing the diaphragm to
the lateral pleural wall. The chest often can be closed without drainage (Figs. 43, 44).

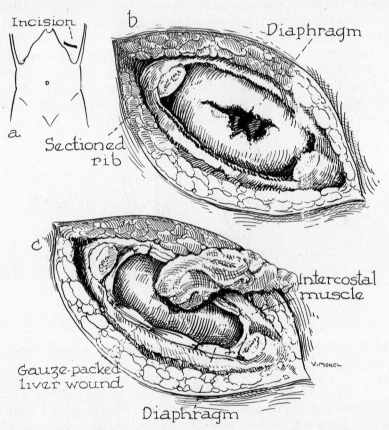

Fig. 43.—Transpleural-transdiaphragmatic exposure and packing of a wound
of the liver following resection of a rib. This approach to the liver usually should
be employed only when there is an already existing, fairly extensive thoracic
wound.

When the wound is on the *left side* and the point of entrance is
below the *eighth rib,* the lesion within the abdomen is likely to be the
more serious. In this group of cases, the abdomen should receive attention first, through a separate incision. If the thoracic injury warrants
exploration, this can be done through an intercostal space.

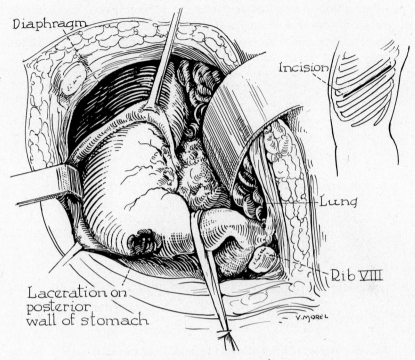

Fig. 44.—Transpleural-transdiaphragmatic exposure of a wound in the fundic portion of the stomach.

Diaphragmatic Injuries

Injuries to the diaphragm can be caused either by a projectile, by a fractured rib, or by blunt force. The diaphragmatic wound may be punctate; it may be a short, linear tear or split; or there may be a large irregular opening. The sloping, muscular portion of the diaphragm is a frequent site of an injury which often involves only that part in contact with the thoracic wall. In about 10 per cent of the cases, herniated abdominal viscera will be found in the thorax, the omentum being the structure most often present. Even when other abdominal viscera are extruded into the thorax, the omentum usually accompanies them. Next in order of frequency of displacement into the thorax are the spleen, the stomach and the transverse colon. Practically all herniations occur through a wound in the left side of the diaphragm. Through and through wounds involving both sides of the diaphragm are seldom encountered, for most of the patients who have such wounds die before they can be transported even to a mobile surgical unit or its equivalent.

5

Interruption of conduction along the phrenic nerve, by injection of procaine or alcohol, or by crushing, dividing, or avulsing the nerve, facilitates repair of the diaphragm and additionally assures continued integrity of the suture line (Fig. 45).

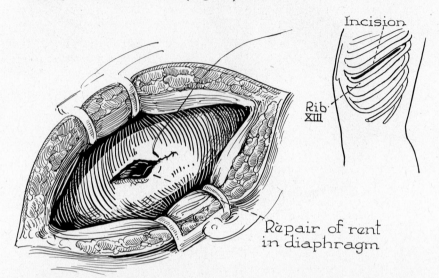

Fig. 45.—Repair of the diaphragm by means of interrupted sutures. The incision is made through the seventh or eighth intercostal space, or a portion of the seventh or eighth rib can be resected. Crushing of the phrenic nerve is often a desirable supplementary procedure, as it facilitates introduction of the sutures and reduces tension along the suture line.

Mortality Associated with Abdominothoracic Injuries

Deaths following abdominothoracic injuries are usually due to the abdominal lesions. The mortality rate is increased when a hollow abdominal viscus has been penetrated. An analysis of a series of cases encountered in the war of 1914–1918 showed that the total operative mortality accompanying abdominal wounds, excluding abdominothoracic wounds, was 49 per cent, while that of abdominothoracic wounds was 55.5 per cent. It has been observed that this difference is not large when it is remembered that thoracic wounds alone resulted in a mortality of about 22 per cent within the period before evacuation to a base. To illustrate what improved methods of managing abdominothoracic wounds can accomplish, in 1916 only 18 per cent of the patients were saved but in November, 1917, the rate of recovery was 49 per cent. In the autumn of 1918, the survival rate reached 66.6 per cent and, in the experience of some surgeons, the rate of recovery was 80 per cent.

REFERENCES

1. Babcock, W. W.: Surgical Affections of the Pancreas. S. Clin. North America. *15:* 101–115 (Feb.), 1935.
2. Bywaters, E. G. L., and Beall, D.: Crush Injuries with Impairment of Renal Function. Brit. M. J. *1:* 427–432 (Mar. 22), 1941.
3. Cathelin, F.: Blessures de guerre de la vessie. Lyon chir. *15:* 109–136, 1918.
4. Devine, Hugh: Operation on a Defunctioned Distal Colon. Surgery. *3:* 165–194 (Feb.), 1938.
5. Dunn, J. S., and Drummond, Hamilton: Ulceration of the Colon in the Neighbourhood of Gunshot Wounds. Brit. J. Surg. *5:* 59–65 (July), 1917.
6. Duval, Pierre: Les plaies thoraco-abdominales. Arch. de méd. et pharm. mil. *69:* 355, 1918.
7. Fullerton, Andrew: Observations on Bladder Injury in Warfare. Brit. J. Surg. *6:* 24–56, 1918.
8. Gage, Mimo, and Ochsner, Alton: The Prevention of Ischemic Gangrene following Surgical Operations upon the Major Peripheral Arteries by Chemical Section of the Cervicodorsal and Lumbar Sympathetics. Ann. Surg. *112:* 938–959 (Nov.), 1940.
9. Gordon-Taylor, Gordon: Cited before.
10. Matas, Rudolph: Endo-aneurismorrhaphy. Surg., Gynec. and Obst. *30:* 456–459 (May), 1920.
11. Prey, Duval, and Foster, J. M., Jr.: Gunshot Wounds of the Abdomen: a Review of Twenty-two Cases. Ann. Surg. *99:* 265–270 (Feb.), 1934.
12. Pringle, J. H.: Cited before.
13. Smith, H. P.: Cited before.
14. Storck, Ambrose H.: Cited before.
15. The Medical Department of the United States Army in the World War. Cited before.
16. Von Haberer, H.: Vascular Surgery in Time of War. München. med. Wchnschr. *87:* 849–851 (Aug. 9), 1940.
17. Wallace, Cuthbert: Cited before.
18. Whipple, A. O.: Surgical Treatment of Carcinoma of the Ampullary Region and Head of the Pancreas. Am. J. Surg. *40:* 260–263 (Apr.), 1938.

CHAPTER IX

POSTOPERATIVE TREATMENT

PATIENTS with abdominal injuries are often more seriously ill following celiotomy than before operation. *Operative trauma, exposure, chilling, loss of blood,* and *anesthesia* combine to increase *shock,* so that supportive treatment following operation is often even more necessary than during the preoperative period. Postoperative care is essentially the same as that preceding and during operation but treatment includes that not only for shock and hemorrhage, but for ileus, peritonitis, and other complications such as wound infection.

SHOCK, HEMORRHAGE, AND HYPOPROTEINEMIA

General Measures

A heat tent should be placed over the abdomen and lower extremities, not only to prevent ileus but also to reduce the incidence of thrombophlebitis or phlebothrombosis in the thighs and legs. When gastric or intestinal contents have spilled into the peritoneal cavity, the patient should be placed in *Fowler's position* following operation unless, on account of shock, *elevation of the foot* of the bed is advisable for a period of from two to twelve hours or longer. *Morphine* sulfate (¼ to ½ grain or 0.016 to 0.032 gm.) should be administered, not only to relieve pain and to insure rest but for the tone stimulating effect which this drug has on the intestine. Ordinarily, ¼ grain (0.016 gm.) of morphine sulfate should be given every four hours unless the respiratory rate becomes less than 12 per minute.

Transfusion of Blood and Plasma

Postoperative *transfusion* of either fresh or preserved whole blood or plasma, or of a solution of dried plasma, is frequently necessary. When intestinal ileus exists, transfusions of plasma are needed for replacement of the amounts of this blood constituent which have passed into the distended loops. If clinical laboratory facilities permit, administration of whole blood, plasma, or serum should be based on estimations of the specific gravity of the blood and determinations of mean corpuscular volume. Not only is maintenance of blood proteins at or near normal essential for sound wound healing, but a deficiency of plasma protein can cause edema or even complete luminal occlusion at sites where stomas have been made, or where repair has been done along the gastro-intestinal tract. The possibilities of maintaining nitrogen equilibrium by parenteral administration of either human or bovine serum albumin or of essential amino acids are being investigated, and the encouraging results so far indicate that, in the future, employment of these substances for the maintenance of protein nutrition may be possible.

Oxygen Therapy

Administration by inhalation of *100 per cent oxygen,* or of a mixture of *oxygen and helium,* is effective not only for the treatment of shock but for removing nitrogen from the distended intestine. Oxygen can be administered efficiently by intranasal catheter or by an oxygen mask, either of which simple methods is more adaptable to military practice than is employment of an oxygen tent. Oxygen, or oxygen and helium, given under positive pressure (6 cm. of water) will relieve pulmonary edema and, when administered at atmospheric pressure, these gases are efficacious in combating anoxemia and cerebral edema. Uninterrupted maintenance of a very high alveolar concentration of oxygen for a long period, however, produces undesirable effects, including pulmonary edema.

Stimulant Drugs

Postoperative administration of stimulant drugs, such as *epinephrine, ephedrine, pituitary extract, caffeine sodium benzoate, pentamethylenetetrazol (metrazol),* 25 per cent solution of pyridine betacarboxylic acid diethylamide (*coramine*), or *alpha-lobeline* may seem necessary, but these substances are usually ineffective. It is ordinarily best to depend on transfusions of large amounts of whole blood or blood plasma or on *infusions,* for combating shock.

DEHYDRATION AND DEMINERALIZATION

Infusions of 5 per cent solution of *glucose, saline* solution, or lactated *Ringer's* solution should be administered. usually in amounts no less than 3000 cc. every twenty-four hours, until fluids can be taken by mouth. These fluids may be given intermittently or by continuous intravenous drip. The temperature of the infused solutions need not be maintained at or above body temperature for, if given at a sufficiently slow rate, no ill effects follow administration of even a cold solution. Because of the ileus-producing effect of glucose, infusion of a solution of glucose in a concentration of more than 5 per cent is to be avoided unless 1 unit of insulin is added to the solution as a buffer for each 2.5 gm. of glucose in excess of the amount necessary to make a 5 per cent solution. The use of *suprarenal cortical extract* not only is of value in restoring blood volume and combating shock, but it also helps to maintain glycogenesis and favorably influences renal function and the distribution of water and electrolytes.

ILEUS

Immediate postoperative introduction of a *gastroduodenal catheter* attached to a *suction* apparatus is ordinarily effective in preventing, as well as in treating, postoperative ileus. The patient may take fluids while the catheter is in place, and it should not be removed until a normal pyloric balance has been established. Postoperative intestinal obstruction, particularly when it is of the "water-hose kink" variety, may often be relieved by the use of the Miller-Abbott tube.

The postoperative administration of drugs which stimulate intestinal tone, such as *prostigmine methyl sulfate,** or *eserine,* for the prophylaxis or treatment of ileus, usually is not necessary. *Pituitary extract* ordinarily not only is ineffective in preventing or relieving adynamic ileus, but may even reduce intestinal tone.

Enemas and *flushes* not only are dangerous in cases in which the large intestine has been injured, but do not relieve distention of the small intestine and, by exhausting the patient and increasing distention of the large bowel, are actually detrimental.

WOUND INFECTION AND PERITONITIS

When there has been extensive damage of the abdominal wall or serious wound contamination, postoperative administration of polyvalent *serum* against the toxins of anaerobic micro-organisms is sometimes advisable, especially if thoroughly satisfactory épluchage cannot be accomplished.

Postoperative administration of sulfonamide drugs may be necessary to supplement the amounts of these drugs which have been introduced into wounds or into the peritoneal cavity at the time of operation.

If wounds are contaminated or infected with anaerobic or facultative anaerobic organisms, such as the micro-aerophilic hemolytic streptococcus, *zinc peroxide* paste is effective. Treatment with this

* Prostigmine is a proprietary preparation, of which the formula is $C_{13}H_{22}O_6N_2S$.

preparation can be started immediately following operation in conjunction with delayed closure of the wound or, if treatment is delayed until signs of infection have appeared, the wound must be reopened widely.

AVITAMINOSIS

The role of vitamins in healing of wounds, in resistance to infection, and in maintenance of hepatic function makes the parenteral or oral administration of concentrated vitamins an important element in the postoperative treatment of patients with wounds of the abdomen. Five hundred to 1000 mg. of *ascorbic acid* should be given every twenty-four hours, along with *vitamin B₁* in doses of from 5 to 10 mg. daily. When an intestinal fistula exists, additional vitamin therapy may be advisable including *riboflavin* (2 mg. or more daily), *nicotinic acid* (25 to 100 mg. daily), or *nicotinic acid amide* (100 mg. daily either by mouth or parenterally).

PULMONARY LESIONS

Postoperative pulmonary complications, especially *atelectasis* and *pneumonitis* are to be anticipated, and an attempt made to prevent them by means of breathing exercises, early mobilization, adequate hydration, and prevention of chilling. Mucus which has accumulated along the air passages during anesthesia should be removed by means of suction. Should pulmonary complications develop in spite of these precautions, bronchoscopic removal of plugs of mucus may be necessary, and if pneumonitis ensues, treatment with sulfonamide drugs and serum must be supplemented by administration of oxygen and by general supportive measures.

THROMBOSIS AND EMBOLISM

Measures for prevention of postoperative thrombosis and embolism, especially *phlebothrombosis* and *thrombophlebitis* in the lower extremities, to be instituted immediately following operation, include adequate hydration, early mobilization, and coverage of the lower extremities by the heat tent which is placed over the abdomen. Postoperative heparinization may rarely be advisable as an additional means of preventing vascular complications following operation.

REFERENCES

1. Altshuler, S. S., Hensel, Hilda M., and Sahyun, Melville: Maintenance of Nitrogen Equilibrium of Amino Acids Administered Parenterally. Am. J. M. Sc. *200:* 239–244 (Aug.), 1940.

2. Best, C. H., and Solandt, D. Y.: Cited before.
3. Boothby, W. M., Mayo, C. W., and Lovelace, W. R., II.: Cited before.
4. Bullowa, J. S. M., Osgood, E. E., Bukantz, S. C., and Brownlee, Inez E.: The Effect of Sulfapyridine Alone and with Serum on Pneumococcic Pneumonia and on Pneumococcus-infected Marrow Cultures. Am. J. M. Sc. *199:* 364–380 (Mar.), 1940.
5. Elman, Robert: Parenteral Replacement of Protein with the Amino-acids of hydrolyzed Casein. Ann. Surg. *112:* 594–602 (Oct.), 1940.
6. Harkins, H. N.: Cited before.
7. Kekwick, A., Marriott, H. L., Maycock, W. d'A., and Whitby, L. E. H.: Cited before.
8. Kendall, E. C.: The Function of the Adrenal Cortex. J. A. M. A. *116:* 2394–2398 (May), 1941.
9. Ochsner, Alton, Gage, I. M., and Cutting, R. A.: The Value of Drugs in the Relief of Ileus; an Experimental Study. Arch. Surg. *21:* 924–958 (Dec.), 1930.
10. Osgood, E. E. (with the technical assistance of Julia Joski): Effectiveness of Neoarsphenamine, Sulfanilamide, Sulfapyridine in Marrow Cultures with Staphylococci and Alpha Streptococci. Proc. Soc. Exper. Biol. and Med. *42:* 795–797 (Dec.), 1939.
11. Paine, J. R., Lynn, David, and Keys, Ancel: Observations on the Effects of the Prolonged Administration of High Oxygen Concentration to Dogs. J. Thoracic Surg. *11:* 151–168 (Dec.), 1941.
12. Paul, J. T., and Limarzi, L. R.: Toxic and Therapeutic Response of Blood and Marrow to Sulfanilamide. Proc. Soc. Exper. Biol. and Med. *43:* 29–32 (Jan.), 1940.
13. Ravdin, I. S., Rhoads, J. E., and Lockwood, J. S.: The Use of Sulfanilamide in the Treatment of Peritonitis Associated with Appendicitis. Ann. Surg. *111:* 53–63 (Jan.), 1940.
14. Scudder, John: Cited before.
15. Storck, Ambrose H.: The Diagnosis and Treatment of Acute Intestinal Ileus. Mississippi Doctor, pp. 30–34, May, 1935.
16. Vorhaus, M. C.: Hypervitamin Therapy in Surgical Practice. Am. J. Surg. *42:* 350–355 (Nov.), 1938.

CHAPTER X

COMPLICATIONS

CLASSIFICATION

COMPLICATIONS of abdominal injuries include those which occur simultaneously with the abdominal wound, and those which develop either shortly thereafter or following a considerable lapse of time.

I. Those incurred simultaneously with the abdominal injury.

    A. Injuries of the head, neck, thorax, spinal column, and extremities due to projectiles or other mechanical forces, including blast injuries of the lungs and tympanic membranes.

    B. Shock and hemorrhage.

    C. Retroperitoneal hematomas.

    D. Contamination of wounds with soil, pieces of clothing, and so on.

    E. Burns, caused either by incendiary bombs, flame throwers, or by the heat of projectiles.

    F. Injuries to the skin, mucous membranes, lungs, or eyes, due to gas or other chemicals.

II. Those occurring subsequent to the abdominal injury.

    A. Early complications (within first twenty-four hours).

        1. Shock and hemorrhage.

        2. Results of exposure to cold and wet.

        3. Peritonitis, including bile peritonitis.

        4. Adynamic ileus, including that due to retroperitoneal hematomas.

        5. Pulmonary atelectasis.

        6. Gas-bacillus infection.

        7. Mental aberrations and psychoses.

    B. Late complications (after twenty-four hours).

        1. Delayed shock and secondary hemorrhage.

        2. Peritonitis, including bile peritonitis.

3. Adynamic ileus, including that due to retroperitoneal hematomas.
4. Mechanical ileus.
5. Thoracic complications:
   (a) Pulmonary atelectasis.
   (b) Pneumonia.
   (c) Pulmonary abscess.
   (d) Empyema.
6. Dehydration.
7. Demineralization and disturbed acid-base equilibrium.
8. Hypoproteinemia.
9. Vitamin deficiency.
10. Thrombophlebitis and phlebothrombosis.
11. Arterial thrombosis, embolism, and aneurysm.
12. Septicemia.
13. Retroperitoneal sepsis.
14. Secondary anemia.
15. Wound infection:
    (a) Tetanus, gas-bacillus, and other anaerobic infections.
    (b) Aerobic pyogenic infections.
    (c) Mycotic infections.
16. Residual abscesses:
    (a) Subphrenic.
    (b) Subhepatic.
    (c) Rectovesical pouch.
    (d) Iliac fossa.
    (e) Perirenal.
    (f) Miscellaneous.
17. Wound rupture.
18. Diaphragmatic hernia.
19. Sinuses due to retained missiles, clothing, or other foreign bodies.
20. Erosion of blood vessels, pleura, or viscera by retained or "wandering" missiles.
21. Intestinal and urinary fistulas.
22. Infection of urinary tract.
23. Traumatic pseudocysts of the pancreas.
24. Mental aberrations or psychoses.
25. Crystalluria, toxemia, and hepatic necrosis due to sulfonamide drugs.

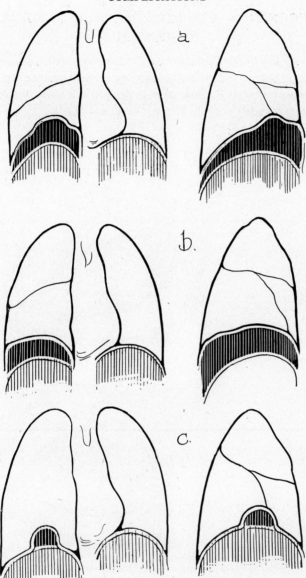

Fig. 46.—Schematic representation of the roentgenologic findings in various types of subphrenic suppuration and in abscess of the liver. *a*, Typical findings when subdiaphragmatic suppuration is secondary to hepatic abscess: obliteration of the cardiophrenic angle in the postero-anterior view, and of the anterior costophrenic angle in the lateral view; *b*, typical findings when subdiaphragmatic suppuration is due to more or less diffuse peritonitis from various causes: obliteration of the costophrenic (instead of the cardiophrenic) angle in the postero-anterior view and of the posterior costophrenic (instead of the anterior costophrenic) angle in the lateral view; *c*, typical findings in the presence of an hepatic abscess which has not ruptured into the subphrenic space.

RECOGNITION AND TREATMENT OF RESIDUAL ABSCESSES

The early recognition of abscesses in the rectovesical space, and of subphrenic and other residual abscesses, by clinical and roentgenologic examinations, followed by adequate drainage, will avert many of the fatalities due to such complications (Figs. 46–51).

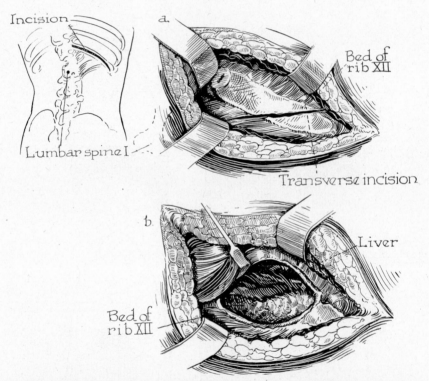

Fig. 47.—The method of approaching the posterior subphrenic space for draining abscesses in that region. After the twelfth rib has been resected, a transverse incision, a, extending across the bed of the rib and through the serratus posterior inferior muscle, the lumbar fascia, and the diaphragm, is made at the level of the spinous process of the first lumbar vertebra. This exposes the liver, b.

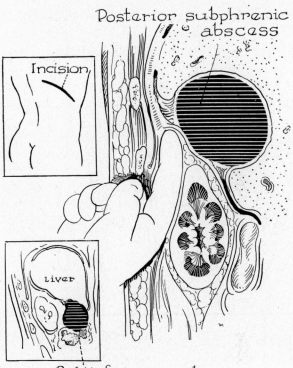

Posterior subphrenic abscess

Incision

Liver

Right inferior space abscess

Fig. 48.—Peeling away the peritoneum from the under surface of the diaphragm overlying an abscess in the posterior superior subphrenic space. After the presence of the abscess has been confirmed by aspiration of pus through a hollow needle, the peritoneum is ruptured, and rubber tissue drains are then introduced. An abscess of the right inferior space can be drained simultaneously through the same incision.

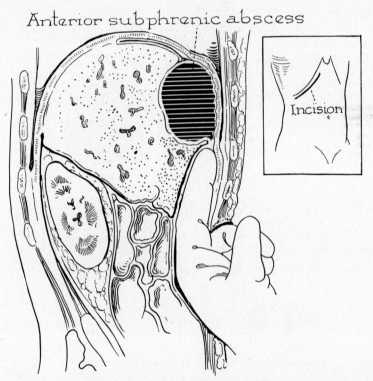

Anterior subphrenic abscess

Incision

Fig. 49.—Method of draining an abscess of the right anterior subphrenic region. Through the subcostal incision indicated in the inset, after an opening has been made through the flat abdominal muscles and the transversalis fascia, the peritoneum is digitally separated from the under surface of the diaphragm until the region of the abscess is reached. After the existence of the abscess has been confirmed by means of aspiration with a hollow needle, the abscess is opened widely, and rubber tissue drains are then introduced.

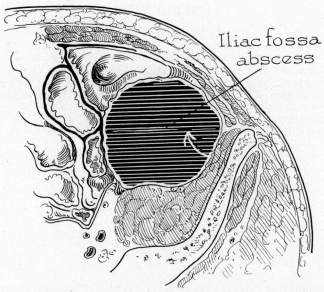

Fig. 50.—A residual abscess of the iliac fossa. Such an abscess usually can be drained satisfactorily through a grid-iron, muscle-splitting incision through the overlying anterior abdominal wall. Soft rubber tissue drains are then introduced and allowed to project through the unclosed wound.

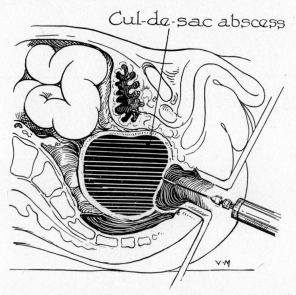

Fig. 51.—Exploratory aspiration of a residual abscess located in the recto-vesical space. After confirming the presence of pus, the abscess is widely opened by spreading scissors or a pair of forceps which has been plunged into the abscess. Rubber tissue drains are then introduced.

REFERENCES

1. Gordon-Taylor, Gordon: Cited before:

2. Granger, Amedee: Cited before.

3. Hartzell, J. B.: The Treatment of Fistulas of the Small Intestine. Surg., Gynec. and Obst. *66:* 108–116 (Mar.), 1938.

4. Jackson, H. C., and Coller, F. A.: Cited before.

5. Jordan, E. P., and Halperin, George: Tetanus Toxoid for Prophylaxis. War Med. *1:* 227–246 (Mar.), 1941.

6. Macnaughton, E. A.: The Treatment of External Fistulas of the Proximal Small Bowel: a Means of Temporary Mechanical Anastomosis. Surgery. *9:* 372–380 (Mar.), 1941.

7. Ochsner, Alton, and Murray, Samuel: Appendicitis. Am. J. Surg. *46:* 566–584 (Dec.), 1939.

8. Storck, Ambrose H.: Complications of Abdominal Traumas. Surg. Gynec. and Obst. *73:* 303 (Oct.), 1941.

CHAPTER XI

RESULTS, MORTALITY, AND STATISTICS

MORTALITY statistics based on patients who reach a hospital are not an index of the total mortality of abdominal injuries of warfare, since many of the injured do not live long enough to be transported to a hospital unit. Because of the demand for attention to the non-fatally wounded casualties, necropsy is seldom made on the bodies of men killed on the field or aboard ship, or even on many of those who die in a hospital. Therefore, much information concerning the character of the abdominal wounds and the associated injuries in fatal cases is unavailable.

The character of military operations, problems of transportation, variations in the types of missiles, and other factors determine mortality results, not only in various periods of a war but even in different divisions of the same forces. Furthermore, the number of deaths following abdominal injury is so much affected by the terrain or the size of a ship, and the medical equipment and personnel, that statistics concerning mortality in various theaters of action are often not comparable.

In the war of 1914–1918 patients with injuries of the abdomen constituted approximately 3.3 per cent of all patients who reached an organized surgical formation. It has been calculated that 10 per cent of the 1,185,000 deaths on the battlefield were caused by the shock and hemorrhage of penetrating abdominal wounds.

In a report on the general surgical experiences of the recent Spanish Civil War, the following observations were made:

1. Of 500 well-recorded abdominal wounds, 239, or 47 per cent, were regarded as inoperable and celiotomy was not performed because:

   (a) The patients were in an apparently hopeless condition. In this group there were 192 patients of whom 97 per cent died.

   (b) The visceral lesions were limited to the liver and it was thought that there was a better chance of survival without operation. This group of patients who were not

129

subjected to operation numbered forty-seven and the mortality was 19 per cent.

2. Celiotomy was performed for penetrating gunshot wounds on 261 patients, 52 per cent of the 500 admissions, on an average of seven and one-half hours after the injury had been inflicted. The lesions of twenty-two of these celiotomized patients, involved almost exclusively the parenchymatous organs, especially the liver. Of this group of 261 patients, 47 per cent recovered.

3. Celiotomy was performed 240 times for lesions of the gastro-intestinal tract, alone or conjointly with other visceral wounds. In this group, only 25 per cent of the patients recovered.

4. Not included in the entire 500 cases were twenty-two in which exploratory celiotomy was performed for penetrating or non-penetrating, uncomplicated visceral injuries. The mortality in this group was 55 per cent. In addition, there were sixteen patients with possibly penetrating, but seemingly uncomplicated, wounds among whom mortality was only 6 per cent.

5. Despite the best care and skill, the mortality associated with exploratory celiotomy was still high: 37 per cent.

6. In spite of the use of transfusions of large amounts of whole or preserved blood, and even under the most favorable conditions for operation, the mortality attending perforating wounds of the gastro-intestinal tract remained high: 75 per cent. The mortality associated with gunshot wounds of the abdomen involving the gastro-intestinal tract, was relatively little improved in comparison with the mortality associated with the same wounds as recorded in the experience of the allied French, British and American surgeons, or of German surgeons, at the close of the war of 1914–1918.

7. Exposure in freezing temperatures, starvation, delay in transportation of patients and hasty organization of surgical staffs in mobile wars exercise decided influence on prognosis. All of these factors were well exemplified at Teruel, the Ebro, Segre, and the Pyrenean slopes.

At the time of the evacuation of the British Expeditionary Force from the continent of Europe in the present war there were, among 2000 patients in hospitals, only about a dozen with injuries of the abdomen or chest, thus attesting to the high mortality currently associated with such injuries.

Since abdominal injuries sustained in modern warfare continue to be so highly fatal, consideration must be given to every available method for the prevention of such wounds and for prophylaxis against the complications which accompany or follow them. The requirements of patients with abdominal wounds demand the co-ordination and co-operation of all military and civilian facilities concerned with their management.

REFERENCES

1. Baron, A. G.: Immediate Results Obtained in the Field Hospitals at the Front, in the Treatment of Penetrating and Complicated Abdominal War Wounds. Rev. españ. de med. y cir. 2: 213–224, 1939.
2. Naegeli, T.: Ueber Bauchkriegsverletzungen. Schweiz. med. Wchnschr. 70: 894–896 (Sept.), 1940.
3. Porritt, A. E.: Discussion of paper by Walker, K. M.: Proc. Roy. Soc. Med. 33: 607, 1940.
4. Walker, K. M.: The Protection of the Soldier in Warfare. Cited before.

GENITO-URINARY INJURIES

GENITO-URINARY INJURIES

Prepared and Edited by the Subcommittee on Urology of the Committee on Surgery of the Division of Medical Sciences of the National Research Council

HERMAN L. KRETSCHMER, *Chairman*

WILLIAM F. BRAASCH

FRANK HINMAN

HOMER G. HAMER

OSWALD S. LOWSLEY

ALBERT J. SCHOLL

With Contributions By

Clark M. Johnson

H. M. Weyrauch

CONTENTS

CHAPTER I   PAGE

PRELIMINARY SURVEY OF THE DIAGNOSIS OF WAR INJURIES OF
    THE GENITO-URINARY TRACT IN GENERAL 135
    Injury to Kidney 135
    Rupture of Bladder 141
    Extraperitoneal Wounds of Bladder or Urethra 143
    Rupture of Urethra 144
    Straddle Injuries of Urethra 145
    Fracture of Pelvis 145
    Infection of Urinary Tract 146
    Incrusted Cystitis 148
    References 148

CHAPTER II

INJURIES OF THE KIDNEY AND URETER 149
    Gunshot Wounds of the Kidney 149
    Crushing Injury and Renal Failure 163
    Gunshot Wounds of the Ureter 166
    Summary 169
    References 171

CHAPTER III

WAR INJURIES OF THE BLADDER 173
    Wounds 173
    Rupture 175
    Operative Treatment 181

CHAPTER IV

CARE OF THE NEUROGENIC BLADDER 187

CHAPTER V

INJURIES OF PENIS AND URETHRA, OF SCROTUM AND CONTENTS,
    AND OF PROSTATE GLAND AND SEMINAL VESICLES ... 203
    The Penis 203

                                                                   PAGE
The Urethra 205
The Scrotum 211
The Testicles in General 211
Luxation of Testicle 213
Epididymo-orchitis or Traumatic Epididymitis 213
The Vas Deferens 214
The Prostate Gland and Seminal Vesicles 214
References 214

                          CHAPTER VI

DO'S AND DON'T'S 217
The Kidney: Nontraumatic 217
The Kidney: Traumatic 218
The Ureter 220
The Bladder in General 221
The Neurogenic Bladder 222
The Lower Tract 222

GENITO-URINARY INJURIES

PRELIMINARY SURVEY OF THE DIAGNOSIS OF WAR INJURIES OF THE GENITO-URINARY TRACT IN GENERAL*

WILLIAM F. BRAASCH, M.D.

INJURY to the urinary tract incurred in war is so often closely concerned with injuries to the surrounding tissues that its recognition may be difficult. An exact diagnosis can be made in many cases only at hospitals which are equipped with instruments of precision employed in urologic diagnosis. At the front the element of shock and the lack of adequate facilities are such that only the simpler methods of diagnosis can be employed. Careful examination for *external evidence* of injury to the kidney, bladder, and urethra should be a routine procedure. The insertion of a urethral catheter, with careful aseptic precautions, may be indicated when the patient is unable to void urine freely, or in order to determine the existence of residual urine and of hematuria which otherwise might not be obvious. In the course of surgical procedures for intra-abdominal lesions, careful inspection for evidence of injury to the kidney, ureter, and bladder should be a routine procedure. When the patient is brought to a hospital where a careful diagnosis is possible, many of the diagnostic measures which are employed in civilian life can be made available. A brief review of procedures which will lead to the diagnosis of traumatic lesions in the urinary tract will follow. Although many of these procedures will be encountered again in following chapters, it is believed that a preliminary survey of diagnosis, in one chapter, will be of service to the user of the manual.

INJURY TO KIDNEY

Renal injuries can be divided into two general groups; namely, penetrating and subparietal. *Penetrating injuries,* which frequently are observed in war, almost always are associated with injury to other organs and tissues. They require immediate surgical care. *Subparietal injuries* usually are confined to the renal cortex, although the renal

* See also the sections on diagnosis contained in the various other chapters.

pedicle and ureter also may be involved. Renal injury sustained by a fall of short distance, from a light blow, or from concussion may consist of a limited cortical rupture of the kidney and may be of no serious consequence.

Symptoms

With a limited rupture of the renal substance the local symptoms may be so slight that the only sign of injury is slight *hematuria,* which may be only microscopic. In many of these cases the hematuria is self-limiting and there is a moderate degree of pain referred to the lumbar region or the lateral portion of the abdomen. In some instances the hematuria may be severe and continue for several days, with the formation of blood clots. The clots may be of such size and

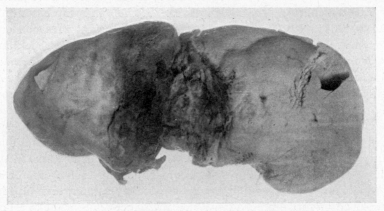

Fig. 1.—Rupture of kidney involving renal pelvis and pedicle (Priestley and Pilcher, Am. J. Surg., May, 1938).

texture that they occlude the renal pelvis or ureter and cause severe renal colic. Clots may accumulate in the bladder so as to fill it completely and cause retention of urine. If the latter complication takes place, there may be some difficulty in differentiating rupture involving the bladder from that involving the kidney. In order to evacuate the clotted blood it is best to employ a large suction syringe attached to a large urethral catheter or to a cystoscope. The bladder having been freed from blood clots, cystoscopic examination may be necessary to determine the nature and extent of the lesion.

Pain referred to the affected renal region may be slight, with mild injury, but when the renal pelvis is blocked by injury or by clotted blood, it may be severe. Perirenal *extravasation* of blood or urine may follow renal injury and cause abdominal pain and tenderness. Abdominal pain and tenderness may be caused also by traumatic peritonism which subsides after a few hours. When the renal pedicle is ruptured (Fig. 1), it is followed by extensive extravasation of blood and urine into the perirenal tissues. There may be little or no blood in the urine which is voided. The presence of clear urine under such conditions would not exclude the possibility of severe renal damage. In case of injury to other organs, the abdominal pain usually will increase in severity.

Methods of Diagnosis

Careful Physical Examination.—Often physical examination will give evidence of multiple abdominal injuries involving other organs and the patient may be in shock, so that any attempt at diagnosis other than surgical exploration would be ill advised. Profound shock suggests coincident injury of the intra-abdominal organs and tissues or extensive intraperitoneal hemorrhage.

Abdominal Palpation.—With extravasation of blood or urine from the ruptured kidney an irregular, diffuse mass often can be felt in the region of the affected kidney. The extent of the perirenal mass varies with the degree of extravasation, but it may not be indicative of the degree of injury. It usually is not particularly painful on pressure unless there is contusion of the perirenal and soft parts, or secondary infection results. The region of hemorrhagic extravasation usually is limited by the perirenal fascia; but if there is an intraperitoneal tear, the hemorrhage may fill the abdomen and become fatal.

Examination of Urine.—Usually this reveals gross blood, although with limited subparietal injury the hematuria may be only microscopic or even absent. Oliguria or retention of urine often is observed with severe renal injury.

Examination of Blood.—The renal function, as indicated by an estimate of the concentration of urea in the blood, usually will remain normal unless there is disease in the other kidney or bilateral renal injury. Estimation of the value for hemoglobin and counting the erythrocytes may indicate the degree of blood loss. Increasing anemia and pulse count are indicative of a concealed hemorrhage. A high leukocyte count may precede other evidences of secondary infection. A variable degree of fever usually accompanies extensive extravasation.

Cystoscopic Examination.—Cystoscopic examination sometimes is indicated to exclude injury to the bladder. It will be necessary in order to carry out retrograde pyelography if indicated. It is also indicated in cases of renal injury in which healing does not occur.

Urography.—Urography usually is available only in establishments to the rear. Surgical intervention often is necessary long before it can be employed. When urography is available, however, it can be of value not alone in determining the existence of a renal or vesical injury but, of greater importance, in determining its extent. The *excretory urogram* may be unsatisfactory when the patient is suffering from shock because of the difficulty in preparation and because of inadequate renal secretion. Perirenal extravasation of blood or urine may obliterate the renal outline and cause a diffuse area of

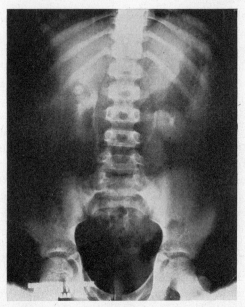

Fig. 2.—Intravenous urogram made two years following renal rupture of the left kidney. Upper calices of the left kidney are obliterated, and only the lower calix and flattened pelvis remain. It is assumed that the upper portion of the kidney is destroyed. Cicatricial caudad displacement of left kidney. Right kidney normal and hypertrophied (Priestley and Pilcher: Am. J. Surg., May, 1938).

perirenal density in the plain roentgenogram. Failure of visualization of the renal pelvis indicates the existence of renal injury but not its degree. In doubtful cases this failure of visualization may be the only evidence of rupture of the kidney. The extent of the renal injury is best determined by means of the *retrograde pyelogram*. The danger attending this method of examination has been exaggerated. When employed with aseptic precautions and with sterile, nonirritating contrast media, no complications should result.

Whichever method is used, the *extent of the injury* usually can

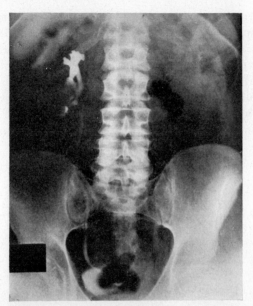

Fig. 3.—Right pyelogram taken six months after injury. There is deformity in the lower calix characterized by irregular extension into the parenchyma and evidence of (1) renal torsion, Grade 2, and (2) cicatricial dilatation of the proximal portion of the ureter (Priestley and Pilcher: Am. J. Surg., May, 1938).

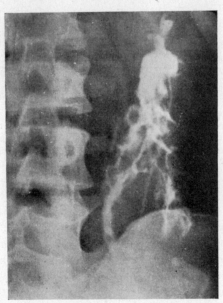

Fig. 4.—Retrograde pyelogram made shortly after injury to kidney. Rotation of kidney, together with extensive extravasation of iodide into perirenal tissue, can be seen (Braasch: Urography).

6

be inferred from the type and degree of deformity visualized. With a slight cortical tear no deformity may be present. In other cases slight deformity of one or more calices or a localized area of sacculation extending beyond the calices may be demonstrated by roentgenologic methods (Figs. 2, 3). If the renal injury is extensive, a diffuse, irregular area may extend over a variable portion of the parenchyma and into the perirenal areas. With a tear in the pelvis the injected medium may be seen extending in all directions from

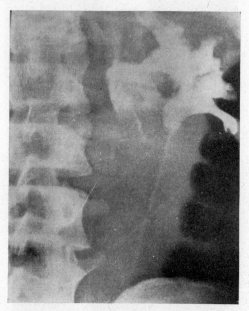

Fig. 5.—Same case as Fig. 4. Pyelogram made several weeks after injury. Rotation is less apparent, although there is marked irregularity and diffuse dilatation of upper major calix, which suggests a bifid type of pelvis in which the injury had been confined more or less to the upper pole of the kidney (Braasch: Urography).

the pelvis and ureteropelvic juncture (Fig. 4). Blood clots often will change the picture by causing bizarre filling defects. A perirenal lesion which has been called "pseudohydronephrosis" occasionally is visualized in the urogram. This consists of a perirenal collection of urine which communicates with the renal pelvis and periodically empties through the sinus.

The subsequent *healing process* may also be visualized by noting the gradual obliteration of the deformity, with resumption of the normal pelvic outline (Figs. 5, 6). If there is considerable damage to one pole, the affected calices and portion of the pelvis may show abbreviation or obliteration. It is remarkable to what extent the pelvis may resume its former normal outline after extensive renal laceration.

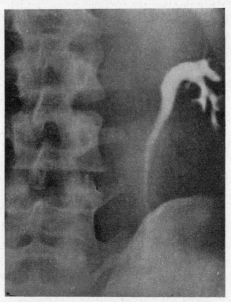

Fig. 6.—Same case as Figs. 4 and 5. Pyelogram made several months after injury. Pelvis appears small and regular, and the upper major calix is absent. The terminal irregularities of the minor calices are well retained (Braasch: Urography).

The urogram also may be of value in determining the position of a *foreign body* relative to the kidney or ureter.

RUPTURE OF BLADDER

Rupture of the bladder may be either *extraperitoneal* or *intraperitoneal,* and occasionally both types occur simultaneously. Establishment of a correct diagnosis may be difficult, since the clinical symptoms often are masked or atypical. In most cases there are multiple injuries involving other structures, and the clinical condition is so obscured by shock and intestinal distention that differential diagnosis may be impossible.

Symptoms

Intraperitoneal Rupture.—The common early symptoms of intraperitoneal rupture are (1) a desire to void with inability to do so, (2) pain, rigidity, and tenderness over the lower part of the abdomen, and (3) evidence of shock. If micturition is possible, it will be painful and frequent and the urine will be stained with blood. Fecal matter may be present in the voided urine in a case of intestinal fistulas. Abdominal distention, rigidity, and tenderness increase with extravasation of urine. Symptoms of peritonitis usually develop soon after injury.

Extraperitoneal Rupture.—Symptoms referable to the urinary tract with extraperitoneal rupture may be very few during the first six or eight hours or more after injury. When pain develops, it may be localized in the suprapubic region or referred to the perineum or penis. Failure to pass any urine is always suggestive of rupture of the bladder when injury of the kidney or urethra can be excluded. On the other hand, rupture of the bladder can be present and the patient experience no great difficulty in voiding. A diminished stream, with difficulty in urinating, might be present with rupture of either the bladder or the urethra. The path of extravasation of urine usually is postperitoneal and extends either toward the renal fossae or into the most dependent part of the extravesical space. If the rupture occurs in association with fracture of the pelvis, symptoms of the latter may mask the possible presence of vesical injury. Early exploratory operation is indicated in all cases in which the diagnosis is doubtful.

Methods of Diagnosis

Abdominal Palpation.—Evidence suggestive of rupture of the bladder may be obtained by abdominal palpation, although generalized abdominal tenderness with distention and shock may obscure the diagnosis. With extraperitoneal rupture a palpable mass can be felt on bimanual examination, extending either to the right or left of the symphysis. Dulness on percussion and induration of the suprapubic tissues can be caused either by overdistention of the bladder or by extravasation of urine. Distention of the bladder may be difficult to determine by palpation of the lower part of the abdomen. It can be recognized on rectal palpation.

Catheterization.—Introduction of a catheter in order to determine the presence and the amount of urine in the bladder is not without danger, but if carefully employed, with aseptic technic, and if chemotherapy is administered previously and subsequently, the possibility of secondary infection will be diminished greatly. Several ounces of urine may be present, even with extensive rupture of the bladder. The retained urine may be clear or only slightly hemorrhagic. In occasional cases the site of perforation may be covered temporarily by omentum so that the bladder does not empty.

Injection of Fluid.—The use of a measured amount of fluid injected into the bladder and withdrawn in order to determine the amount retained is a time-honored method. This procedure, however, carries with it a considerable risk of peritoneal infection, and the information it gives may be misleading.

Examination of Blood.—This may give data of definite value. The leukocyte count and sedimentation rate may be increased, even when infectious complications are not present. Determination of nonprotein nitrogen often is of considerable value, although evidence of reduced renal function would not be conclusive when accompanied by severe injury in other structures.

Rectal Examination.—This is of little value in most cases of rupture of the bladder. Its greatest value is in determining the presence of an overdistended bladder.

Excretory Urography.—An excretory urogram visualizing the outline of the bladder, as well as the kidneys and ureters, carries with it less danger and greater accuracy than any other method. Unfortunately, this method is possible only when the patient's general condition permits and when roentgenographic facilities are available. It will be difficult to prepare for urographic examination patients who are in shock, and usually too they will be unable to excrete sufficient iodine to visualize the vesical, ureteral, or renal outlines in the urogram.

Retrograde Cystography.—When available, the site and extent of the rupture in the bladder may be outlined. The cystogram can be made either by injecting sterile gas or air into the bladder, or by injecting nonirritating solutions of organic iodides.

Cystoscopic Examination.—If other methods fail to exclude the possibility of rupture, cystoscopy may be tried. Hematuria may be profuse, and clots may be present so that inspection is difficult. The existence of foreign bodies in the bladder, such as missiles, fragments of bone, or soft calculi, can be determined in no other way.

Suprapubic Exploration.—In cases of abdominal injury, a suprapubic incision will enable the surgeon to determine the condition present in doubtful cases. *Early exploratory operation is indicated in all cases in which the diagnosis is in doubt.*

EXTRAPERITONEAL WOUNDS OF BLADDER OR URETHRA

Wounds of the bladder or deep urethra rarely exist independently. Wounds of the buttocks, thighs, or hips, and sacral and perineal wounds involving the rectum without evidence of abdominal disturbance, may be related to extraperitoneal rupture of the bladder or urethra and should always be investigated carefully. All patients who have such wounds should be catheterized, with care and with aseptic precautions, if there is any difficulty in voiding urine. *Hematuria,* when present, would give a valuable hint. When the rectum and bladder are both injured, the urine usually will contain *feces* as well as blood. Urine and blood may drain from the external wounds. Signs of *urinary extravasation* usually are present and follow the path of least resistance, which is along the most damaged fascial planes.

RUPTURE OF URETHRA

Wounds in the posterior urethra present problems similar to wounds of the bladder. The clinical observations will depend largely on whether the rupture of the urethra is anterior or posterior to the triangular ligament. The most common site of rupture is in the bulbous urethra, anterior to the triangular ligament.

Symptoms and Signs

If the rupture is *anterior* to the triangular ligament, the penis, scrotum, and perineum may be swollen and discolored, and the lesion usually can be readily recognized. Extravasation of urine may extend superficially to the abdominal wall. If the rupture is *posterior* to the triangular ligament, swelling and extravasation may not be noticeable on inspection, but they soon extend into the deeper tissues. It may be difficult to determine a minor tear in the posterior urethra. Severe contusion of the perineum may cause clinical symptoms and signs which simulate those of minor injury to the urethra. Difficulty also may arise in differentiating rupture of the posterior urethra from rupture of the bladder.

Chief symptoms of rupture of the urethra, anterior or posterior, are pain in the perineum, bleeding from the meatus, hematoma, and urinary retention. In an occasional case there are no immediate symptoms suggestive of urinary complications. Evidence of profound shock may be present, particularly on rupture of the posterior urethra. Inability to void urine is present in most cases, although occasionally a little blood-tinged urine may be passed after the first attempt to urinate, but not thereafter. When accompanied by fracture of the pelvis and shock, it may be difficult to differentiate rupture of the urethra from that of the bladder. If there is no coincident injury of the bladder, little if any immediate extravasation of urine is likely to occur because of contractural spasm of the internal sphincter which prevents the bladder from emptying. The bladder and urethra may be ruptured at the same time, and failure to recognize the dual injury may result in serious complications. With coincident rupture of the bladder and extravasation of urine, the lower portion of the abdomen becomes rigid and tender.

Diagnostic Procedure

In all severe injuries involving the pelvis and lower part of the abdomen, the *urethral meatus* should be inspected immediately. A bloody ooze is sometimes seen at the meatus, even though no urine is passed. With a history of no voiding after the injury a large globular mass may develop twelve hours later in the suprapubic region as the result of urinary retention. If the patient is unable to void, an attempt should be made, under most careful asepsis, to *pass a catheter* with gentle pressure. If obstruction is encountered in the urethra and if no urine is obtained, or a few drops of bloody urine, it may be assumed that a rupture of the urethra is present. If the catheter passes into the bladder, a partial rupture of the urethra may be present. *If the first attempt at catheterization fails, further efforts should not be made, but plans should be made immediately for surgical intervention.* A simple *rectal examination* often will reveal the rupture with an extravasated mass of blood or urine. When the diagnosis is doubtful, a urethrogram or cystogram made at different angles may be of value in recognizing the condition present.

Rules.—With all severe injuries to the lower portion of the abdomen or pelvis the following rules should be remembered: (1) always examine for a show of blood at the external meatus; (2) if the patient cannot void and rupture of the urethra is not evident, an attempt should be made to pass a catheter, with aseptic precautions; (3) look for other evidence of injury in the lower part of the urinary tract; and (4) do not wait for refined diagnostic aids; if in doubt, exploratory operation and drainage are indicated.

STRADDLE INJURIES OF URETHRA

Symptoms vary from the most trivial to severe with minor degrees of injury. With complete rupture, however, severe pain and tenderness are present with evidence of perineal or scrotal hematoma and, later, extravasation of urine. Shock usually is not so marked as in the group of patients with intrapelvic rupture.

FRACTURE OF PELVIS

Rupture of the urethra and bladder often occurs with fracture of the pelvis and should always be excluded. In fact, rupture of the posterior urethra rarely occurs without fracture of the pelvis. The *clinical signs* usually observed with the combined injury are: (1) inability to move the legs, which are rotated outward; (2) extreme pain on movement; (3) deformity and crepitus; and (4) hematoma in the perineal and scrotal tissues. Injury to the urethra with pelvic fracture occurs more frequently than to the bladder. Unless rupture of the bladder is associated, extravasation of urine does not occur early because of reflex spasm of the sphincter. When the urethra or bladder is ruptured, any of the clinical signs previously described may be present. After fracture of the pelvis and rupture of the urethra or bladder, stones are likely to form as the result of invasion by bacteria with urea-splitting tendencies. Secondary calculi may occur in both kidneys and in the bladder.

INFECTION IN URINARY TRACT

Injury of the urinary tract frequently is complicated by secondary infection, which may become of major clinical importance. Fortunately, modern *chemotherapy* offers a method of treatment which, if intelligently employed, will control the infection in many cases. In order to carry on such treatment it will be essential to determine the type of infecting bacteria, since bacteria respond variously to different chemotherapeutic agents. A comparatively simple *method of identification* is available in the microscopic examination of the urinary sediment stained by the Gram method. This method is also of clinical value in determining the existence of mixed infection.

Identification of Invading Bacteria

For therapeutic purposes it is of practical importance to classify the bacteria as either *bacilli, cocci,* or *streptococci*. Differentiation of bacteria usually is possible from the microscopic appearance and the staining qualities of the various bacteria. *Gram-negative bacilli* are found most frequently in urinary infection. Included among the more common gram-negative bacilli are Escherichia coli, Aerobacter aerogenes, Proteus, Salmonella, and Pseudomonas. The last three groups are the hardest to eradicate. When present they usually cause alkaline urine, as determined by the hydrogen-ion concentration. *Gram-positive cocci* are present much less frequently than the gram-negative bacilli. Micrococci are the most common forms of gram-positive cocci encountered in urinary infections, and usually they are not pathogenic. Staphylococcus aureus, when present, can be a very virulent invader. The most common member of the Streptococcus family in urinary infections is Streptococcus faecalis. It usually is a secondary invader and often is present with mixed infections. It is not as virulent as some of the other streptococci, which, fortunately, are not often encountered. Cultures of the urine may be necessary in some cases in order to determine more exact bacterial differentiation.

Selection of Therapeutic Agent

Having identified the infecting bacteria, it becomes necessary to select the therapeutic agent which fits the case. Bacteria of the Escherichia, Proteus, and Salmonella groups usually can be eliminated by sulfathiazole or mandelic acid. *Mandelic acid* is given in amounts of 6 to 8 gm. daily, divided into four doses. Moreover, the daily intake of fluid is limited to 1200 cc., and the diet is of the high acid ash type. Normal renal function is necessary for adequate secretion of either drug in the urine. An average daily administration of 3 gm. of *sulfathiazole*, divided into three or four doses, should be continued for a period of eight or ten days. With severe infection it may be advisable to employ 4 or 5 gm. daily during the first two or three days. Alkalinization of the urine may increase the bactericidal action of the sulfonamide compounds in some cases. Preparations of mandelic acid usually are combined with an acidifying agent such as ammonium chloride. They are not bacteriostatic unless the *p*H of the urine is maintained at a level of 5.0 or 5.5.

Staphylococci, gonococci, and micrococci are controlled best by sulfathiazole or sulfapyridine. Most streptococci, if present, respond best to sulfanilamide. *Sulfapyridine* and *sulfanilamide* are given in amounts of 3 or 4 gm. daily, divided into four doses. Streptococcus faecalis, however, can be controlled best by administration of mandelic acid combined with drugs such as ammonium chloride, which acidify the urine.

In the use of the sulfonamide compounds the usual precautions are necessary to guard against *systemic reactions* as evidenced by cyanosis, blood dyscrasia, eruptions on the skin, fever, and so forth. Nausea and anorexia usually can be controlled by reduction of dose or temporary cessation of the administration of the drug. Acidosis may result from the administration of mandelic acid if renal function is subnormal.

Irritability of the bladder without infection is a common condition in warfare after exposure to severe, long-continued privation and cold. It may be recognized by the absence of any evidence of bacteria or pus in the urine. The symptoms are largely on a functional basis and usually are relieved by rest in bed.

INCRUSTED CYSTITIS

Infections of the bladder which are secondary to injury frequently are complicated by infection with urea-splitting bacteria, such as the Proteus ammoniae and Pseudomonas. As a result of such infection, deposits of calcium with incrustation of the mucosa of the bladder often occur. This condition can be suspected from the presence of small amounts of calcareous material in the urine and symptoms of severe dysuria, tenesmus, and hematuria. The diagnosis is best established by cystoscopic examination. Chemotherapy, removal of the incrustations with the heel of the cystoscope, acidification of the urine, and topical applications of a 20 per cent solution of silver nitrate to the affected regions are indicated.

REFERENCES

1. Braasch, W. F.: Urography. Philadelphia, W. B. Saunders Company, 1927, pp. 455–457.
2. Keyes, E. L.: Present Status of the Urology of War. J. A. M. A. 71: 323–327 (Aug. 3), 1918.
3. Priestley, J. T., and Pilcher, Frederick, Jr.: Traumatic Lesions of the Kidney. Am. J. Surg. 40: 357–364 (May), 1938.
4. Sargent, J. C.: Injuries of the Kidney with Special Reference to Early and Accurate Diagnosis through Pyelography. J. A. M. A. 115: 822–825 (Sept. 7), 1940.
5. Young, H. H., and Davis, D. M.: Practice of Urology. Philadelphia, W. B. Saunders Company, 1926, pp. 137–181.

CHAPTER II

INJURIES OF THE KIDNEY AND URETER

ALBERT J. SCHOLL, M.D.

GUNSHOT WOUNDS OF THE KIDNEY

GUNSHOT wounds of the kidney, caused by either rifle bullets or shrapnel, are most commonly found in conjunction with more frequent and serious wounds of adjacent viscera, and may be readily overlooked. While injuries of either abdominal or thoracic viscera usually overshadow, and at times divert attention from, the renal lesion, prompt and efficient treatment of the kidney wound may prevent grave disability and possible loss of life in an important group of cases.

Incidence

Statistical reports from different countries vary widely with regard to the incidence of war injuries, but agreement is general concerning the rarity of uncomplicated renal lesions and the high mortality in complicated cases. In a series of 2121 abdominal wounds reported from British hospitals, there were 155 associated injuries to the kidney (7.3 per cent). Of the 155 injuries to the kidney, 69 were uncomplicated. In Laewen's report of 42 gunshot wounds of the kidney, in 37 the abdomen was penetrated, and in only 5 were the injuries extraperitoneal.

Fullerton found the most frequently associated injury in his group to be a wound of the *pleural cavity*. In 17 (40 per cent) of his 42 cases of gunshot wounds of the kidney, the missile reached that organ by way of the thorax. In 7, hemothorax developed, and in 3 empyema. The *liver* also was involved in 14 (33 per cent). The *spine* was injured in 6 (14 per cent), and the *intestine* in 5 (12 per cent).

Pathology

Gunshot injuries of the kidney are classified as wounds of the parenchyma and wounds of the hilum.

Wounds of Parenchyma.—The most common wounds of the renal

149

parenchyma are of the perforating type, although furrows, complete
destruction of either pole, or extensive shattering of the kidney may
occur. A moderate number of parenchymal wounds are slight, especially those in which the edges or poles are injured. When the center of the kidney is injured, the damage is usually severe. The nature
of the projectile has little particular effect on the injury, although
bullet wounds destroy a portion of parenchyma only slightly larger
than the size of the bullet, whereas shrapnel makes a more irregular
wound, and there is greater destruction of tissue. In shrapnel injuries,
the edges of the wound are more likely to be contused, and the adjacent parenchyma may become necrotic on account of arterial injury. Many parenchymal wounds also involve the *calices,* but urinary
extravasation is not usual unless the wound is large and extends into
the pelvis of the kidney itself. If urine escapes from the wound or
surface, it is probable that the *pelvis* or *ureter* has been injured.

Wounds of Hilum.—In wounds involving the hilum, the *renal
artery* or one of its larger branches may be divided. When the renal
artery has been severed, the patient usually dies before reaching the
hospital; when one of the larger branches has been cut through or
obstructed by formation of a clot, nephrectomy is usually resorted to.
Although renal veins anastomose, the arteries do not, and consequently arterial injury, even of the smaller vessels, may cause extensive cortical necrosis.

In an occasional case, the renal vessels are divided, leaving an
intact ureter. Injuries to the *renal pelvis,* like injuries to the renal
artery and veins, are infrequent; though both may be injured by the
same missile. *Peritoneal tears* are common, and intraperitoneal hemorrhage or infiltration of urine into the peritoneal cavity is found in
many cases.

Although the incidence of *minor lacerations* and *contusions* of the
kidney, which are not uncommon in civil life, is probably high in
time of war, they rarely receive treatment, as they are overshadowed
by other lesions or are disregarded by the patient or surgeon. Nevertheless, it is important that the surgeon keep them in mind, because
they may simulate extensive renal damage but rarely require intervention. In some contusions hematuria may be severe; but in the absence of shock, or when there is evidence of perirenal bleeding,
watchful waiting is the most desirable course to follow.

Traumatic rupture of the kidney similar to that occurring in civil
injuries is not infrequently seen, and may be due to transmitted force
or to injuries not related to war wounds.

Symptoms and Diagnosis (see also p. 136 and following)

The location of the wound and the presence of hematuria are the first indications of renal damage in most cases. In uncomplicated renal lesions the patient's general condition is usually good.

Abdominal Wall.—There is partial fixation and rigidity of the abdominal wall, and tenderness on abdominal palpation over the injured kidney and in the corresponding costovertebral region. Rarely is abdominal relaxation sufficient to permit accurate palpation of the renal region, although in some cases extensive perirenal bleeding produces a large mass in the flank which is readily felt through the rigid muscular wall. When the abdomen also has been perforated, usually extensive abdominal rigidity is present, although either partial or generalized abdominal rigidity does not always mean a lesion of the peritoneal cavity. Gunshot wounds of the chest or chest wall, extensive hematoma of the renal region, or intra-abdominal hemorrhage from any condition also can cause abdominal rigidity.

Shock.—Usually, although not always, shock is present. In uncomplicated cases it is generally not severe, and depends to a certain extent on the amount of blood lost. In cases in which an injury to the abdominal viscera, thorax, or spinal column is associated, shock is usually marked. Even in uncomplicated renal injuries, however, *the severity of shock is not always an accurate index of the degree of renal damage.*

Hematuria.—Varying from microscopic amounts to massive hemorrhage, blood is present in the urine in most cases, although the hematuria may not occur immediately. In the early stages it is not excessive, and after several days tends to cease spontaneously. If the wound involves only the parenchyma of the kidney, hematuria may be slight or absent.

It is necessary to make certain that the blood is coming from the kidney and not from the bladder, as the latter is not an infrequent manifestation of associated injury of the spinal cord. In all wounds of the loin, the urine should be examined for microscopic evidence of blood. If necessary, *catheterization* should be done, as retention is common in cases of renal injury and may be due to a concomitant lesion of the spinal cord. Absence of hematuria may be due to division of the ureter, to obstruction of it by blood clots or fragments of renal tissue, or to extensive damage to the renal pelvis.

Secondary hemorrhage into the bladder is fairly frequent, and is most common in the second or third week after injury, but may appear as late as two months afterward. It is not unusual for these late hemorrhages to be so severe that they cause death. Consequently, it is desirable, even in cases in which only slight renal injury is present, to keep the patient absolutely quiet, preferably at rest in bed if possible for at least two weeks after injury. Secondary hemorrhage may be spontaneous, or it may be an exacerbation of persistent primary hemorrhage. Differing from the primary bleeding, it is often accompanied by clotting of blood in the bladder.

Urinary Extravasation.—Urinary extravasation in the renal region is generally not marked, and is usually seen in cases of extensive pelvic or ureteral tears. Urinary infection occurs frequently and early, even when the renal damage is only slight or moderate. In many cases it persists long after renal repair has been established.

Roentgenology.—Roentgenologic examination gives definite diagnostic information relative to the state of the kidney and should be made as soon as the patient reaches the base hospital or its equivalent, as gas distention develops quickly and obscures the renal outline.

PLAIN ROENTGENOGRAM.—A plain roentgenogram of the kidney may be done in the presence of extensive secondary injuries which prohibit more detailed urologic studies. Haziness of the renal outline, obliteration of the psoas margin, or deviation of the spine away from the injury suggests perirenal bleeding.

EXCRETORY UROGRAM.—Rarely will there be time or opportunity for excretory urography in the first few days after trauma, but when possible it is of great assistance. It aids in locating and defining the extent of the injury, and determines the presence and function of the opposite kidney. If a fair concentration of the opaque medium is excreted by the injured kidney, it is probable that the renal injury is slight and early treatment unnecessary. Excretory urography, similar to the plain roentgenogram, can be done in the presence of extensive complications, and even when the patient is unconscious. It has the disadvantage that the secretory powers of the kidney may be inhibited or reduced by trauma, and that in the presence of shock the ability of the kidney to secrete is reduced still further by a drop in blood pressure and lowered volume of blood to the kidney. The injured kidney continues to secrete only as long as the renal tissue and blood supply are still intact. During the period of recovery, the secretory power of the damaged kidney as well as that of the sound contralateral organ is inferior to the immediate post-traumatic ability to secrete. Therefore, in most cases excretory urography performed shortly after rupture gives the most reliable information concerning the gravity of the lesion. There is a group of cases, however, in which early excretory ureteropyelograms are unsatisfactory, and better results may be obtained several days later.

Excretory urography is particularly graphic in cases of minor injury to the kidney, and is usually of more diagnostic assistance in gunshot wounds than in cases of rupture from civil trauma, as gunshot wounds frequently leave a large proportion of the kidney undamaged. In some instances of even fairly extensive tears, sufficient opaque solution is secreted by the remaining normal segment of parenchyma to indicate the extent of damage present.

CYSTOSCOPY, URETERAL CATHETERIZATION, AND RETROGRADE PYELOGRAPHY.—Sometimes these may be necessary to establish the diagnosis, and usually they give much more accurate information than that obtained by excretory urograms. However, lack of time or equipment usually prohibits these procedures in the early days after injury. Moreover, cystoscopy is usually hazardous in the presence of shock or extensive bony lesions. Exacerbation or recurrence of bleeding may occur from shifting the patient's position or, more rarely, from instrumental manipulations. When cystoscopy is indicated and can be carried out, and time and the condition of the patient permit, it should be done.

In the majority of cases of gunshot wounds, particularly those seen in front-line hospitals, the finer points of diagnosis obtainable by cystoscopy are time-consuming and unnecessary. The only immediate questions to be settled are: *Is operative intervention imperative, and is the opposite kidney capable of sustaining life in the event that nephrectomy is obligatory?* The intravenous urogram usually gives a satisfactory answer to both these questions. Physical findings, site of entrance of the projectile, pain, swelling, and hematuria generally determine the diagnosis and the location of the lesion.

In those cases in which satisfactory ureteropyelograms are obtained, the visualized changes in the course of the ureter and the outline of the renal pelvis give accurate information concerning the pathologic changes present. Deviation of the ureteral outline toward the vertebral column, upward displacement of the ureteropelvic juncture, and narrowing of the calices suggest perirenal extravasation.

Treatment

In most cases of gunshot wound, care of the renal condition is less urgent than that of complicating lesions, and in a large number of cases only conservative local treatment is necessary.

Shock.—Renal injury is characterized by hematuria and internal hemorrhage. Shock should be treated symptomatically. In cases in which it is due to renal bleeding, surgical exploration of the kidney is indicated.

Hematuria.—Hematuria, even though marked, is not sufficient reason for early surgical exploration. Primary hematuria usually subsides in from twenty-four to forty-eight hours, but if it persists and is profuse the kidney should be explored.

Exploration. LUMBAR APPROACH.—Urinary extravasation usually calls for early and extensive incision and free drainage of the region. In cases in which it is doubtful whether the abdomen or the renal region should be opened, remember that lumbar incision carries less risk, and if necessary the abdomen can be explored through the same incision (Fig. 7). Explore the renal region first. An adequate lumbar

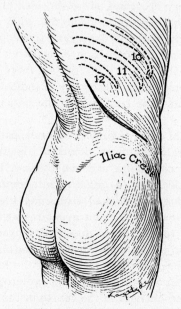

Fig. 7.—Incision for exposure of renal region.

approach permits evacuation of clots, thorough visualization of the kidney, and opens an easily drained region that may be securely packed if necessary. After completing the repair of the kidney, the lower angle of the incision should be elongated transversely, the peritoneum opened in front of the colon, and the adjacent viscera examined, as the peritoneum and its contents are damaged in more than 90 per cent of cases of wounds to the kidney.

ABDOMINAL APPROACH.—In cases in which primary abdominal exploration is performed and renal damage is probable, the kidneys should be palpated. In some cases positive information is obtained by this route; but if injury is present, usually an obscured field due to perirenal bleeding makes it difficult to determine the extent of renal damage even if the posterior layer of peritoneum has been opened over the kidney. Exploration of the renal region *transabdominally* is usually not advisable, as it opens up a poorly drained field, which is readily contaminated from frequently present abdominal infections. If during abdominal exploration a hematoma or obvious renal damage is found, it is unwise to open the posterior peritoneum for either further exploration or evacuation of clots. For the same reason, transabdominal nephrectomy should rarely be done, as it is particularly hazardous and bears a high mortality record. In many cases, fairly large perirenal hematomas need no immediate evacuation. Although they may eventually cause further renal damage and disability, no harm results from delaying their removal until opportunity and the state of the patient make this procedure safe.

EXPLORATION OF RENAL FOSSA.—When conditions found during the course of laparotomy indicate that exploration of the renal fossa is necessary, a second incision should be made, using the lumbar approach. It is, however, preferable to postpone renewed intervention for several days, as this delay provides time for the patient to recover from shock, for his general condition to improve, for diagnostic study to be made, and in most instances for reduction of free hemorrhage in the operative field. On the other hand, early exploration is imperative in cases in which bleeding from the kidney is excessive, although it may have incited considerable shock.

Wounds of Kidney, Liver, and Diaphragm Combined.—Combined wounds of the kidney and liver, although serious, usually require only conservative management, and frequently surgical intervention is neither advisable nor necessary. Wounds of the diaphragm encountered in the course of exploration of the kidney rarely require repair.

Surgical Procedures for Wounds of Kidney

In the treatment of wounds of the kidney, there are three possible surgical procedures: (1) drainage of the renal region, (2) partial nephrectomy and repair of the injured kidney, and (3) nephrectomy.

Drainage of Renal Region.—This permits inspection, evacuation of blood clots, and control of bleeding. It is the simplest procedure, and may be done quickly with only slight risk to the patient. Foreign bodies and fragments of shrapnel should be searched for carefully and removed. All loose fragments of tissue should be taken out. Drainage should be free and plentiful; usually it consists of three or four large *Penrose drains,* either plain or containing gauze wicks. The drains should be placed carefully to reach all parts of the wound. In closing the incision, care should be taken not to suture so tightly that obstruction of drainage results.

Drainage is *indicated* in cases in which time or the condition of the patient has not permitted complete studies to determine the condition of the opposite kidney.

CONTROL OF BLEEDING.—If hemorrhage is encountered, an effort should be made to control it with catgut ties or sutures. In suturing or clamping bleeding points, care should be exercised not to injure the peritoneal contents or the great vessels; on the right side the duodenum lies close to the kidney and is easily damaged. No large segments of tissue should be grasped with toothed forceps, and no extensive or deep suturing should be done without certain knowledge of the involved structures. Usually general oozing does not permit complete localized hemostasis, and is best controlled by *packing* with iodoform or plain gauze. Lumbar incision permits firm packing, and sufficient gauze should be used to control all bleeding. A piece of rubber dam or similar material should be spread in the wound before packing to facilitate removal of the gauze and to prevent recurrence of bleeding when the gauze is taken out. When lacerations of the kidney are severe, and when the patient is in a precarious condition, thorough *packing* controls the hemorrhage until the patient is better able to stand nephrectomy.

When the kidney is not removed and drainage is installed, it should be continued until at least the tenth postoperative day.

Partial Nephrectomy, Renal Repair, and Plastic Operations.— Frequently these procedures are employed with good results in the closed, civilian type of renal rupture, but they are usually unsatisfactory for *infected, penetrative wounds.* This is especially true of soldiers entering the hospital in shock after long periods of exposure. In cases in which partial nephrectomy or suture has been done, parenchymal infection, necrosis, and late bleeding usually necessitate reopening the wound later, and in some cases nephrectomy.

The *control of hemorrhage* usually calls for surgical intervention. A partial nephrectomy is not likely to remove the cause of the bleeding, and a patient already anemic should not be exposed to the risk of a fresh hemorrhage from a sutured or a partly resected organ. Rarely are limited operations justifiable.

Nephrectomy. INDICATIONS.—The kidney should be removed in cases of persistent hematuria, multiple deep lacerations of the parenchyma, or damage to the vascular pedicle. A patient who has rupture involving the entire vascular pedicle rarely reaches the operating table in a condition suitable for operation.

When the ureter is severed, the pelvis torn, or the kidney lacerated and urine is escaping from the wound, results are usually poor unless nephrectomy is done. However, in the presence of a ureteropelvic tear, slight or no infection, and a not unsound kidney, no harm results from the flow of urine over tissues as long as it has a free exit.

Nephrectomy is a simpler procedure than most conservative or repair operations, and usually removes the cause of bleeding. In the small group of cases in which the condition of the patient is satisfactory and the kidney so damaged that ultimate nephrectomy will be necessary, or there is uncontrollable bleeding from the kidney, nephrectomy is the procedure of choice. *Nephrectomy takes less time than a repair, removes a potential field for infection, and limits future bleeding from the operative site.* It also eliminates a secondary operation and the late disability and sequelae which so frequently follow reparative procedures.

EARLY NEPHRECTOMY.—In the early days after injury nephrectomy is difficult and hazardous. Most observers agree that in only rare instances is early nephrectomy indicated or advisable. Increased experience has shown that in many cases in which early nephrectomy would have been employed formerly better results are obtained by efficient drainage; nephrectomy if it is necessary is left until a later date.

INCISION FOR RENAL EXPLORATION.—When renal exploration is necessary, and a wound presumably leading to the kidney is found in the renal region, this wound may be enlarged transversely. The kidney is a difficult organ to deliver, especially when exploration of the pelvis or renal vessels is required. Consequently, renal exploration should not be undertaken through too small an incision. Attempts to deliver a traumatized kidney through a small, poorly placed incision frequently result in further trauma and increased hemorrhage. Therefore, if an incision is to be made, its location and size should be determined on the basis of the best possible exposure. A large, well-placed incision is of further advantage in the control of any emergency condition and the reduction of operating time. Besides, in most cases a large incision heals as readily as a small one.

POSITION OF PATIENT.—A 4-inch strip of adhesive tape passed completely around the hips of the patient and under the operating table will immobilize the patient in the necessary position. Elevation of the kidney rest and moderate breaking and lowering of both ends of the table increase the supra-iliac space, through which the kidney must be approached, and also put tension on the lateral muscles of the body, permitting them to be divided more easily. Fixing the patient in a satisfactory position and keeping him in this position throughout the operation are among the most essential factors in successful surgical intervention, and greatly facilitate the operative procedure (Fig. 8).

TECHNIC OF NEPHRECTOMY.—The *posterolateral incision* permits the best exposure of the kidney and its pedicle, and combines the so-called "posterior and anterior incisions." When the abdomen is to be explored after disposing of the renal condition, the anterior incision may be lengthened, the peritoneum opened in front of the colon, and the abdominal contents examined. The posterolateral incision sacrifices a minimum of muscles, vessels, and nerves. It may vary from a crescentic curve to one in which a definite angle is formed between its upper and lower parts. The lower part of the incision starts midway between the anterior crest of the ilium and the last rib, passing backward almost parallel to the iliac crest until it crosses the border of the

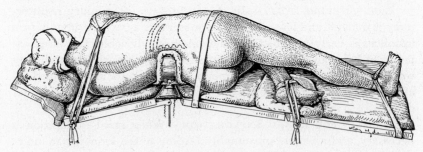

Fig. 8.—Position of patient for kidney operation. Strap over hip is adhesive tape, 2 inches wide.

latissimus dorsi muscle, where it turns upward to end in the angle between the last rib and the spinal column.

After the skin and subcutaneous tissue have been cut through and pushed back, the superficial layer of muscles is seen, anteriorly the *external oblique,* posteriorly the *latissimus dorsi* (Fig. 9). The external and internal oblique muscles are cut through in the part presenting in the incision. The anterior border of the latissimus dorsi is also cut through. The *fascia overlying the erector spinae muscles* is cut through well into the upper angle of the incision. This permits the skin and subcutaneous tissues to open up more freely. The *transversalis fascia* is then split in a small area, which brings into view the *renal capsule* and usually the underlying clots. The opening into the transversalis fascia is then spread with the fingers, bringing the renal region into view (Figs. 10, 11, 12).

In the average case it is not necessary to cut the erector spinae muscles or the underlying *quadratus lumborum*, although no apparent postoperative difficulty results if this is done. The *first lumbar nerve* usually passes down on the lateral portion of the quadratus lum-

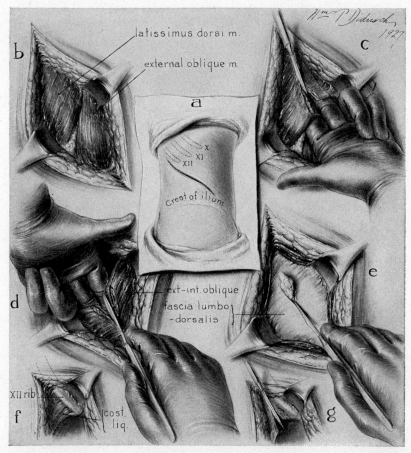

Fig. 9.—Extraperitoneal lumbar nephrectomy. *a*, Skin incision, extending parallel with the twelfth rib and about 2 cm. below it, downward and forward to a point above the crest of the ilium; *b*, the latissimus dorsi and external oblique muscles are exposed, showing Petit's triangle; *c*, cutting the latissimus dorsi muscle; *d*, dividing the external and internal oblique muscles; *e*, incising the lumbodorsalis fascia. The retroperitoneal fat protrudes through the incision; *f*, exposing the costovertebral ligament; *g*, dividing the costovertebral ligament (Lowsley and Kirwin: Clinical Urology. Williams and Wilkins Co.).

borum, and should be protected from injury. The *twelfth intercostal nerve* and its lateral cutaneous branch come out just below the twelfth rib, and usually parallel the upper angle of the incision. If possible, it is advisable to retract these nerves out of the incision, although cutting them, in spite of being followed by disagreeable anesthesia, usually

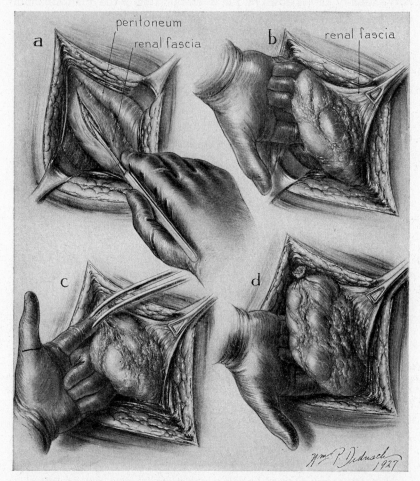

Fig. 10.—Extraperitoneal lumbar nephrectomy. *a,* Incising the perirenal fascia (Gerota's capsule); *b,* anterior and lateral freeing of the kidney from the surrounding adipose tissue by sharp and blunt dissection; *c,* clamping adhesions and freeing the upper pole. The likelihood of encountering aberrant blood vessels must be kept in mind when freeing the poles of the kidney. The poles should be freed very cautiously, the tissues being carefully examined before they are cut; *d,* freeing the lower pole (Lowsley and Kirwin: Clinical Urology. Williams and Wilkins Co.).

causes no permanent difficulty. If greater visibility is necessary, the *last costovertebral ligament* may be cut, which permits the *twelfth rib* to be pulled well up out of the incision. This rib may be forcibly

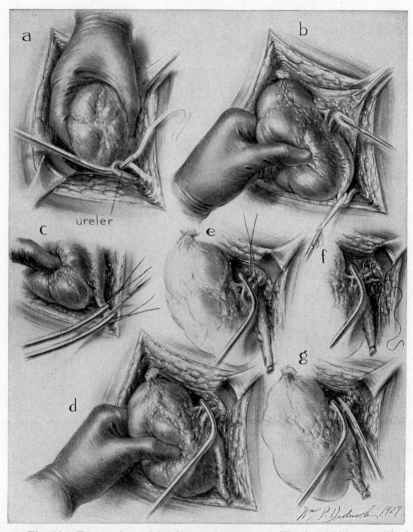

ureter

Fig. 11.—Extraperitoneal lumbar nephrectomy. *a,* The freed kidney is lifted
up, the ureter located, and a tape passed beneath it to facilitate its handling; *b,*
dissecting the perirenal fat from the vascular pedicle; *c,* the ureter is then
divided between clamps and ligated; *d,* showing the vascular pedicle with the
first clamp applied; *e,* the second clamp applied and the first clamp removed;
first ligature being placed around the portion of the pedicle crushed by the first
clamp; *f,* the renal pedicle, with two ligatures applied and a transfixion suture
about to be placed; *g,* dividing the pedicle (Lowsley and Kirwin: Clinical Urology. Williams and Wilkins Co.).

pulled up, and if it is cracked or broken more operative space is
obtained and no particular harm is done.

In cases in which a rudimentary twelfth rib is present, an abnormality recognized by a preliminary roentgenogram, it is necessary to

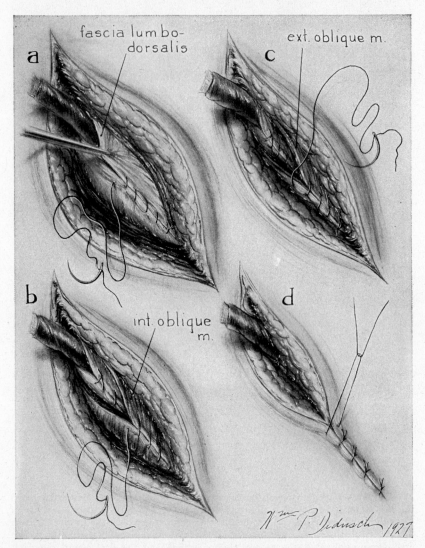

Fig. 12.—Extraperitoneal lumbar nephrectomy. *a,* Suturing the lumbodorsalis fascia; drain in place; *b* and *c,* suturing the internal and external oblique muscles; *d,* suturing the skin (Lowsley and Kirwin: Clinical Urology. Williams and Wilkins Co.).

remember that the *pleura* usually comes down below the eleventh rib. Consequently, the incision in the presence of a rudimentary twelfth rib should be placed considerably below the eleventh rib in order to avoid injury to the pleura.

CRUSHING INJURY AND RENAL FAILURE

Crushing injury to the limbs, with extensive destruction of the muscles, may result in marked or fatal suppression of renal function. This condition is found most commonly in association with injuries in air raids, especially among civilians who are crushed and pinned for hours under the debris of bombed houses. Cases also have been reported in which the condition has resulted from accidents to members of mechanized forces and among workers in civil industries.

Reports of the condition have been few and most of them have been published recently. Bywaters, in a report before the Royal Society of Medicine, stated that the Medical Research Council had collected details of more than seventy cases. He stated that the condition was recognized in Germany during the war of 1914–1918, that it was mentioned in official books on military surgery, and that histologic aspects of the condition were discussed. Reports seem not to have appeared in English since 1923, in spite of the fact that the injury does occur in civil practice, as has been said.

Clinical Course

In most of the cases the patients have sustained crushing injury such as that which might result from being buried, with beams or fallen masonry pressing on their arms or legs. The duration of the crushing has varied greatly. Robertson and Mathews stated that there does not appear to be any direct relationship between the duration of the crushing and the seriousness of the subsequent condition. As far as records seem to disclose, the shortest period of crushing to be followed by the development of the crush syndrome has been forty-five minutes; the case was reported by Belsey. The longest recorded period of crushing to be followed by the crush syndrome, according to Robertson and Mathews, was twenty-six hours. The average period is about eight to ten hours.

Belsey described the following changes which take place in the crushed limb. Necrosis of muscle occurs; it is patchy in distribution and may not correspond to damaged areas of the overlying skin, such as would suggest that the necrosis was due to direct pressure. There is edema of the limb and increase of tension in the tissues within the fascial compartments. Loss of nerve function has been recorded in the majority of cases and commonly has involved all the nerves of the limb, a distribution suggesting that the failure of conduction is due to ischemia and asphyxia rather than to direct pressure.

There is usually moderate shock at the onset, which apparently is controlled by the usual measures, but which reappears after a period of from a few hours to several days. Bywaters stated that, during the initial phase, hemoconcentration occurs from loss of plasma into the injured part, which becomes swollen and hard. There is also loss of sensation and power. Wheals, and later blisters, appear on the skin; arterial pulsation may be impaired distally. The secondary phase of shock usually requires more vigorous treatment, such as intravenous administration of fluids or transfusion of blood.

The patient usually looks critically ill, even after the symptoms of shock have abated. The volume of urine is low and the specific gravity becomes fixed at about 1.015. The urine is bloodstained and contains pigmented casts in the early stages. Later there is a tendency for the urine to become clear and less in quantity. The blood pressure rises and the patients usually have the symptoms of uremia.

The concentration of blood urea, phosphate, and potassium increases; the carbon dioxide combining power of the blood drops. Muscular twitchings occur, the patient becomes drowsy, edema increases, and death may occur about the seventh day.

Unquestionably the renal function of many patients who sustain crushing injuries undergoes only slight interference. In some cases the condition is completely overlooked; in others the patients recover without any definite treatment. It has been observed in general that urinals are rarely called for by air-raid casualties. Riddell remarked on the need for careful examination in order not to overlook the early crush syndrome. The telltale wheals, or simply localized erythema of the skin, will draw attention to the lesion. The only hope of cure is in early recognition.

Pathology

The pathologic findings have been well discussed by Bywaters, Robertson and Mathews, and others.

Muscle necrosis is the one etiologic factor common to all these cases. Bywaters described three types of muscular lesions:

1. Only part of the muscle is necrotic, and there is a sharp boundary line between living and dead tissue, corresponding exactly with the pressure marks seen on the skin. This is the commonest type of change and is probably due to ischemia from direct pressure.

2. The whole muscle may be necrotic, irrespective of areas of

pressure on the skin. These muscles are contained within tight fascial sheaths, and it seems probable that rise of intrafascial pressure may be responsible for the ischemic necrosis that is seen.

3. Necrosis of isolated muscle fibers is found.

The *kidneys* are large and swollen. Microscopically the collecting tubules contain many pigment casts similar to those found in the urine. The casts are composed of brownish or greenish granular blood pigment, mixed with necrotic epithelial cells and pus cells. There is also severe tubular damage to the distal convoluted tubules and to the loops of Henle, often with complete necrosis, discharge of hyaline casts into the interstitial tissue and surrounding cellular reaction.

Prognosis

The prognosis is usually good if patients survive the critical period of seven or eight days. In fatal cases, death usually comes rather suddenly on the seventh to ninth day. In about a third of the reported cases the patients have recovered; most of them were less critically injured primarily than those who died. Patients injured so severely that circulation to the limb is not reestablished also are likely to recover. The extent of the renal lesion is indicated by the rise in concentration of blood urea and in blood pressure. Bywaters stated that in the fatal cases the urea curve is a straight line which rises until the patient dies on or about the seventh day. If patients survive, the curve may be as has been described and then fall, or it may fail to rise so much and fall earlier. Increase in output of urine, decrease in amount of edema, and reduction of hypertension suggest that the critical stage has been passed and that recovery is probable. Survival of the patient usually is followed by return to normal of the affected limb, although cases in which late amputation was necessary owing to pain, paralysis, or destruction of muscle have been reported.

Treatment

Recognition that crushing injuries may be followed by renal failure makes it essential to institute immediate measures for prevention of this fatal complication. Recovery is rare if hypertension and oliguria have appeared. The first consideration should be treatment of the renal failure. Bywaters advised establishment of good alkaline diuresis as soon, and as rapidly, as possible, even before treatment of the shock or of the local lesion. After renal failure has occurred, intravenous administration of fluids and diuretic drugs is of little value; usually it only increases the edema.

A number of surgical procedures, such as amputation and wide incision through the crushed tissue, and decapsulation of the kidneys, has been reported. As yet the number of patients treated surgically has been few, and the results inconclusive.

Prevention of renal obstruction by early administration of fluid, including alkalis, apparently offers the greatest chance of success. Robertson and Mathews reviewed reports of a number of cases in which the patients recovered and in which success was attributed to administration of alkalis. The rationale of treatment with alkalis is based on two facts: (1) These patients all present marked acidosis. (2) It is probable that the pigment found in these cases is precipitated in the tubules, if the urine is acid; if the urine is alkaline, the pigment will pass through without renal injury.

Various alkalis have been used. Blackburn and Kay gave 1000 cc. of 2 per cent solution of sodium bicarbonate rectally on the fifth day after injury; on the eighth day they started oral administration of sodium bicarbonate, giving a total of 96 grains (6.4 gm.) in seven days. Longland and Murray administered 360 grains (24 gm.) of potassium citrate by mouth daily for four days and 480 cc. of 3.3 per cent solution of sodium sulfate intravenously on the third of these days before the urine became alkaline. Henderson gave 540 cc. of 3.3 per cent solution of sodium sulfate intravenously daily for four days.

GUNSHOT WOUNDS OF THE URETER

The ureter is only rarely injured by gunshot wounds. It is small, well protected by heavy bony structures and, because of its flexibility, is usually pushed aside by the missile and sustains only minor injuries. It is so closely related to many important structures that when it is injured, other organs are usually damaged also. Rarely does uncomplicated ureteral injury occur which would permit early surgical attack directed primarily toward ureteral repair. The ureteral injury is most commonly secondary and is discovered during abdominal exploration for other injuries.

Diagnosis

Injury to the ureter is characterized by *urinary leakage* either into the peritoneal cavity, into the surrounding tissues, or, if the tract of the missile remains open, onto the skin. Shifting fascial planes or adhesions may obliterate the tract of the bullet and result in extravasation of urine into the surrounding tissues and tumefaction.

Hematuria may occur after a minor injury to the ureter, rarely with complete severance, and is more commonly considered a symptom of renal damage than of ureteral injury.

In the presence of *peritoneal fluid* after a gunshot wound of the abdomen, urinary leakage should be suspected and, if demonstrated, the ureter examined for injury. Lack of recognition of the ureteral or pelvic source of the abdominal fluid usually results in abdominal fistula or more rarely peritonitis.

With complete severance of the ureter, *obstruction* is encountered on ureteral catheterization. Urographic studies may indicate the lesion and the path of the urine although, when extravasation is present, diffusion of the contrast medium is not unlike that seen in cases of rupture of the kidney.

Intravenously injected *indigocarmine* will determine whether urine is present in the drainage from the wound.

Treatment

Drainage of any urinary accumulation is the most important immediate treatment.

Lateral Ureteral Injuries and Incomplete Tears.—These have a tendency to close spontaneously, and simple drainage of the region may be sufficient. A retained ureteral catheter, which should be changed frequently, aids in restoring the ureteral channel.

Complete Severance.—In cases of complete severance of the ureter without infection, *anastomosis* of the severed ends or *reimplantation* of the ureter into the pelvis or bladder (Fig. 13) is possible, but rarely practical. In the majority of cases delay, hemorrhage, infection, and extensive trauma with destruction of a segment of the ureter render plastic repair impossible. Several cases have been reported in which the wounds occurred in civil practice and were treated directly after injury. When this had been done, in some the immediate results appeared favorable, but almost invariably the late results proved unsatisfactory.

If the opposite kidney is adequate, and no obvious infection is present, *ligation of the ureteral stump* is justifiable. Next to simple drainage of the field, this is the easiest, least shocking procedure. Silk should be used, and the stump dropped back into the wound. When infection is present in the kidney, and the patient's condition permits, *nephrectomy* (p. 156) should be done. If the condition of the opposite kidney is unknown, simple ureterostomy, pelviostomy, or nephrostomy can be done.

Persistent Fistula.—Nephrectomy is usually necessary for persistent urinary fistula. Sufficient time should be allowed for spontaneous closure, during which period diagnostic cystoscopic procedures may be carried out. Nephrectomy done under these circumstances, with the patient in an improved general condition, carries much less risk than when it is done in the early days following injury.

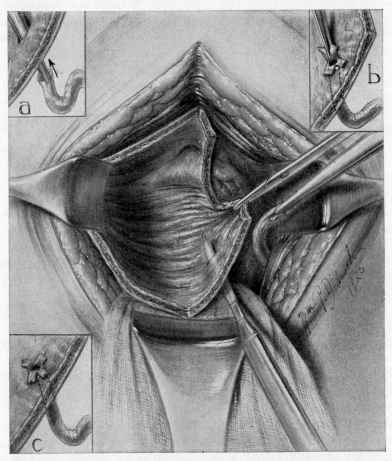

Fig. 13.—Reimplantation of ureter into bladder following resection of a portion of the bladder. In this case, the right ureteral orifice was removed and the ureter severed about 1 inch (about 2.5 cm.) above the bladder wall. A stab wound is made obliquely through the bladder wall. *a,* The ureter is then drawn through the stab wound; *b,* splitting the end of the ureter; *c,* showing the ureter sutured to the bladder wall (Lowsley and Kirwin: Clinical Urology. Williams and Wilkins Co.).

Extravasation.—Tissues in which extravasation has occurred should be incised widely. When extravasation occurs in the flank, a posterolateral incision should be made which permits satisfactory drainage as well as examination of the upper part of the ureter, renal pelvis, and body of the kidney.

Lower Ureteral Injury.—Wounds of the middle and lower segments of the ureter are usually associated with abdominal injuries, and are found in the course of abdominal exploration. In the rare instances in which exploration of the lower half of the ureter is indicated, it is best exposed by a *straight incision* parallel to the outer border of the rectus muscle or by a *muscle-splitting incision.* This incision is made through the outer portion of the rectus muscle, or the muscle may be retracted to the midline and the incision passed down at its distal margin. The incision should be of ample length and carried directly down to the pubic bone. After the muscle and fascial bands have been penetrated, the peritoneum is retracted toward the midline, and usually the ureter is carried with it. Careful blunt dissection should be done with the fingers. Not infrequently in cases of trauma to the ureter it will be found that the peritoneum is also damaged, or it may be injured in retracting it toward the midline. Any peritoneal tears should be repaired as soon as they are discovered. The lower part of the ureter lies deep in the incision and is difficult to locate, especially when the periureteral tissues have been distorted by the path of the missile.

Upper Ureteral Injury.—Injuries of the upper part of the ureter are usually found on exploration of the kidney and renal pelvis. A posterolateral incision gives the best exposure of this region.

SUMMARY

1. Examine the urine in all cases in which there is possibility of trauma to the kidney. If necessary catheterize the bladder to obtain a specimen.

2. Urinary retention is frequent in cases of renal injury; watch for overdistention of the bladder.

3. Plain roentgenograms and excretory urograms should be taken as early as possible.

4. Many penetrative wounds of the kidney require no treatment; exploration of the renal region should be done only when there is excessive hematuria—persistent or recurrent—free perirenal bleeding is present, or extensive renal damage is suspected.

5. In cases of combined wounds of the kidney and abdomen the renal injury is usually secondary and the abdominal injury demands the more urgent treatment. In case of doubt as to

which region should be explored first, explore the renal region. Exploration of this region carries less risk, and the incision can be easily lengthened to permit exploration of the abdomen (see also paragraph 10).

6. If, in the course of an abdominal operation, perirenal hematoma is found which requires evacuation, this may be done extra-peritoneally. If renal exploration is essential, it can be done through a posterolateral incision, preferably several days later.

7. Transabdominal exploration of the renal region is not advisable; transperitoneal nephrectomy is particularly fatal.

8. In front-line hospitals the simplest operative procedures are usually the safest and most likely to permit the ultimate survival of the patient.

9. The three most common surgical procedures are drainage, nephrectomy, and plastic repair.

Drainage of the renal region is the most satisfactory early procedure. It is simple, quickly carried out, and permits evacuation of clots, removal of fragments of tissue and foreign bodies, and the packing of the region to control hemorrhage. Drainage should be free and the wound closed in the usual manner. Secondary operation may be done later if necessary when the patient is better able to stand an extensive procedure.

Nephrectomy is reserved for cases in which urgent removal of the kidney is essential, such as persistent excessive hemorrhage, extensive destruction of the vascular pedicle, and in cases in which the kidney is completely shattered.

Plastic repair of the kidney is usually unsatisfactory and is rarely indicated. It is time-consuming, is frequently followed by infection and secondary hemorrhage, and nephrectomy usually is required later. On the other hand, removal of all loose fragments of renal tissue and segments without an adequate blood supply is essential.

10. In exploring the kidney, a posterolateral incision is usually the most satisfactory. It should be ample in length, and, after exploration of the renal region, the lower angle of the incision should be lengthened, the peritoneum opened, and the abdomen explored.

11. Crushing injury to the limbs, with extensive muscular destruction, may result in urinary suppression.

12. Clinical features of crushing injury with renal failure are

edema, tissue tension, and loss of nerve function of the limb; shock; staining of the urine with blood; reduction of urinary volume; rising blood pressure; symptoms of uremia and possibly death about the seventh day after the injury.

13. Pathologic features of crushing injury and renal failure are muscular necrosis; large, swollen kidneys; and damage to the renal tubules.

14. A third of the patients who have undergone crushing injury with renal failure have recovered. Prognosis is good if they survive the critical period of seven or eight days.

15. Treatment of crushing injury and renal failure consists in bringing about early alkaline diuresis. Treatment of the renal failure should precede measures for combating shock.

16. In the presence of peritoneal fluid, leakage of urine should be suspected, and, if demonstrated, the ureter should be examined for injury.

17. The ureter usually sustains only minor injuries which have a tendency to heal spontaneously; unless an emergency exists, early ureteral repair is not necessary.

REFERENCES

1. Belsey, Ronald: Discussion on the Effects on the Kidney of Trauma to Parts Other than the Urinary Tract, Including Crush Syndrome. Proc. Roy. Soc. Med. 35: 328–332 (Mar.), 1942.
2. Blackburn, Guy, and Kay, W. W.: Crush Injuries with Renal Failure and Recovery. Brit. M. J. 2: 475–476 (Oct. 4), 1941.
3. Bywaters, E. G. L.: Discussion on the Effects on the Kidney of Trauma to Parts Other than the Urinary Tract, Including Crush Syndrome. Proc. Roy. Soc. Med. 35: 321–328 (Mar.), 1942.
4. Fraser, J., and Drummond, Hamilton: A Clinical and Experimental Study of Three Hundred Perforating Wounds of the Abdomen. Brit. M. J. 1: 321–330 (Mar. 10), 1917.
5. Fullerton, Andrew: Gunshot Wounds of the Kidney and Ureter as Seen at the Base. Brit. J. Surg. 5: 248–288 (Oct. 1), 1917.
6. Henderson, R. G.: Recovery from Uraemia Following Crush Injury. Brit. M. J. 2: 197 (Aug. 9), 1941.
7. Lockwood, A. L., Kennedy, C. M., and Macfie, R. B.: Observations on the Treatment of Gunshot Wounds of the Abdomen with a Summary of 500 Cases Seen in an Advanced Casualty Clearing Station. Brit. M. J. 1: 317–320 (Mar. 10), 1917.
8. Longland, C. J., and Murray, John: A Case of Recovery from Crush Syndrome. Lancet. 2: 158–159 (Aug. 9), 1941.
9. Riddell, V. H.: Discussion on the Effects on the Kidney of Trauma to Parts Other than the Urinary Tract, Including Crush Syndrome. Proc. Roy. Soc. Med. 35: 334 (Mar.), 1942.
10. Straus, D. C.: Recent Gunshot Wounds of the Kidney: with Report of 4 Cases. S. Clin. North America. 2: 635–681 (June), 1922.

7

11. Robertson, H. R., and Mathews, W. H.: Crush Syndrome. Canad. M. A. J. *46:* 116–120 (Feb.), 1942.

12. Wallace, Cuthbert: A Study of 1200 Cases of Gunshot Wounds of the Abdomen. Brit. J. Surg. *4:* 679–743 (Apr.), 1917.

13. Walters, C. F., Rollinson, H. D., Jordan, A. R., and Banks, A. G.: A Series of 500 Emergency Operations for Abdominal Wounds. Lancet. *1:* 207–213 (Feb. 10), 1917.

CHAPTER III

WAR INJURIES OF THE BLADDER

OSWALD S. LOWSLEY, M.D.

WAR injuries to the bladder include every form of injury encountered in civilian life and others directly connected with combat, such as bullet wounds, bayonet thrusts, shrapnel-fragment wounds, and crushing injuries from accidents in which mechanized units take part. Concerning this subject quotation is freely made from "Clinical Urology" by Lowsley and Kirwin.

Most vesical injuries occur during distention of the bladder, when it rises above the symphysis pubis and becomes an abdominal organ, in which state it is much more subject to trauma.

Injuries to the bladder are of three types: (1) contusions caused by kicks, falls, and so forth; these are seldom diagnosed and are of slight clinical importance, although rarely they may be serious enough to cause death by shock and hemorrhage; (2) wounds, usually communicating with the exterior, caused by puncture or perforation by sharp or blunt objects; and (3) rupture, which is by far the most common injury.

WOUNDS

Etiology

Wounds of the bladder are encountered very infrequently in civil practice, and belong primarily to the realm of war surgery. They are produced chiefly by bullets or by pointed instruments, such as bayonets, knives, or fragments of shell or shrapnel. During the war of 1914–1918 such injuries were fairly frequent and were inflicted as a rule by shrapnel. In civil practice, the bladder is occasionally injured accidentally during surgical operation or urethral instrumentation. Perforation of the vesical wall by a fragment of bone may occur in fracture of the pelvis.

Pathology

Wounds may be slight or extensive, depending on the size of the penetrating object. They may be either *intraperitoneal* or *extraperi-*

173

toneal. The former are more serious as a rule. Vesical wounds associated with injuries to the buttocks, perineum, or thighs are more likely to be extraperitoneal, whereas those inflicted through the abdomen are usually intraperitoneal. Such wounds may be uncomplicated, but usually the surrounding structures are involved to some extent. In war injuries or pelvic fractures, the associated injuries to the neighboring viscera, bones, and large blood vessels may be extensive.

Symptoms (see also pp. 141, 143)

The symptoms and course vary greatly in wounds of the bladder, depending on the extent of the wound, its location (whether intraperitoneal or extraperitoneal), and the associated injuries. *Shock* is likely to be present in some degree, and may be very severe; but cases of serious traumatization have not infrequently been reported in which shock or other early indications of vesical injury were trifling or wholly absent. *Hemorrhage* may be so severe as to prove rapidly fatal, or the detection of blood in the urine which the patient is able to void normally may be the first indication that the bladder has been injured.

The most common *early symptoms* suggestive of injury of the bladder are pain in the hypogastrium, more or less shock, and a constant desire to void and inability to do so, or the passage of a small amount of bloodstained urine. Escape of bloodstained urine through the wound is, of course, conclusive proof of penetration of the bladder. However, the urine may extravasate into the perivesical tissues or leak into the peritoneal cavity. With the intraperitoneal extravasation of urine, the abdomen becomes distended, rigid, and tender, or the urine may extravasate extraperitoneally and form a palpable mass in one or both flanks. If the wound involves the peritoneum, there will be free fluid in the abdominal cavity. These symptoms, however, are not usually in evidence until several hours after the accident.

Diagnosis (see also p. 142)

Early diagnosis and surgical repair are of the utmost importance, since urinary extravasation and subsequent infection are the chief dangers for those patients who survive the initial shock and hemorrhage.

Penetrating wounds of the bladder are always to be suspected in wounds involving the *hypogastrium, buttocks,* or *perineum.* The direction and extent of all such wounds should be studied carefully with the possibility in mind of injury to the bladder and the gravity of such injury when it does occur. In wounds involving the buttocks, particularly, associated extraperitoneal wounds of the bladder have not infrequently wholly escaped discovery. Wounds near the vesical neck are most likely to escape notice because of the difficulty of examining this region with the ordinary cystoscope. If some time has elapsed between the injury and the examination, the swelling and edema, or hemorrhage, may make it impossible to see the wound. In severe injuries, cystoscopy is, of course, impossible.

Sometimes the history and physical examination are sufficient to establish the diagnosis without instrumentation. *Catheterization, cystoscopy,* and *injection cystography* and *aerograms* are all valuable in making the diagnosis and in ascertaining the location and extent of the wound, but their use is always accompanied by the risk of increasing the incidence of infection, and in extensive injuries may be out of the question. *Excretory cystograms* are useful, if sufficient time for this procedure can be allowed and danger of infection is less by this method. All of these methods are considered under the diagnosis of rupture (pp. 142, 179).

Treatment

The treatment consists of supportive measures and surgical repair at the earliest possible moment after the diagnosis has been made, with drainage of the bladder and of the infiltrated tissues if extravasation has occurred.

RUPTURE

Etiology

The usual cause of rupture of the bladder is some *external violence* to an overdistended viscus. *Alcoholism* is one of the most important factors predisposing to rupture of the bladder, since in the intoxicated state the bladder is often subjected to overfilling, and this, together with the associated relaxed condition of the abdominal muscles, renders it more susceptible to injury. Other predisposing causes are *vesical distention* from any cause; chronic conditions (enlarged prostate, urethral stricture) causing *urinary retention;* and *disease of the bladder* (inflammation, ulceration, atony, diverticula; Figs. 14, 15). Spontaneous rupture and rupture from muscular effort have been reported, but invariably in these cases there is some accessory factor, such as overdistention or disease, which has produced weakening of the vesical wall. Rupture of the bladder is frequently associated with *crushing injuries* involving fracture of the pelvis (25 out of 166 cases of fracture, Campbell; 65 out of 169 cases, Bartels). The incidence of such cases in civilian practice is increasing with the increase of automobile accidents; the same may be expected in military practice. Rupture or perforation sometimes occurs from extravesical pathologic processes (Fig. 16).

Occasionally rupture may be secondary to *instrumentation* or *surgical manipulations*. It may occur from overdistention with irrigating fluid at cystoscopy, in which event a pathologic weakening of the wall will usually be found; the wall may be penetrated by the cystoscope,

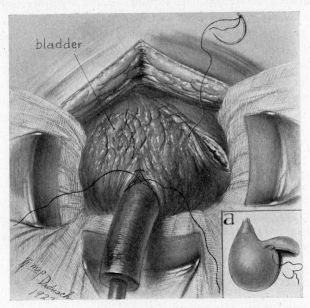

Fig. 14.—Repair of bladder wall after diverticulectomy. (Usually the sac is removed in its entirety and the hiatus in the bladder wall closed with a running catgut suture, but in the case illustrated only partial resection could be done). *Inset a,* Repair of the bladder with the remaining portion of the sac, resulting in obliteration of the neck of the diverticulum and the conversion of the two cavities into one (Lowsley and Kirwin: Clinical Urology. Williams and Wilkins Co.).

lithotrite, or other instrument, or there may be too deep fulguration of a tumor or ulcer. In recent years extraperitoneal ruptures at the vesical orifice, caused by the electrical loop in vesical-neck resection, have been reported.

Pathology

Rupture of the bladder may be either intraperitoneal or extraperitoneal, or may partake of the nature of both classifications.

Intraperitoneal Rupture.—This is more frequent than extraperitoneal rupture, probably because the injury usually is to the anterior abdominal wall and it occurs when the bladder is distended. When the bladder is only partially filled, extraperitoneal rupture is more frequent. The *site* of intraperitoneal rupture is usually on the posterosuperior aspect, which is the least supported and most vulnerable portion of the bladder. Extravasation of urine into the peritoneum rapidly follows, making early surgical intervention imperative.

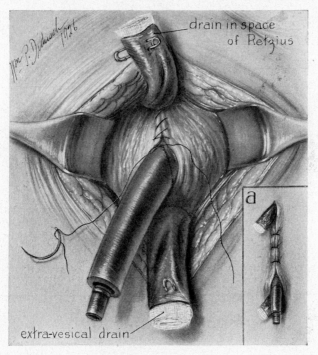

Fig. 15.—Method of placing drainage tube and Penrose drains after removal of a diverticulum; *inset a,* skin closure (Lowsley and Kirwin: Clinical Urology. Williams and Wilkins Co.).

Extraperitoneal Rupture.—This is most likely to occur in conjunction with fracture of the pelvis. It results from severe violence directed against the hypogastrium or perineum, and, when this violence is simultaneously exerted in both these directions, the bladder has small chance of escaping serious injury. The most frequent *site* of extraperitoneal rupture is in the trigon. Occasionally the tear may be in the preperitoneal tissues in front, the prevesical space, or in the side of the vesical neck. With a fracture of the pelvis the bladder may either rupture or, if the bones have been splintered, be perforated in one or more places by fragments of bone. Perforation is more likely to occur with a distended bladder, but may happen also with a comparatively empty one.

Symptoms (see also p. 141)

Both the intraperitoneal and extraperitoneal types of rupture give similar symptoms, but the manifestations in the former type are usu-

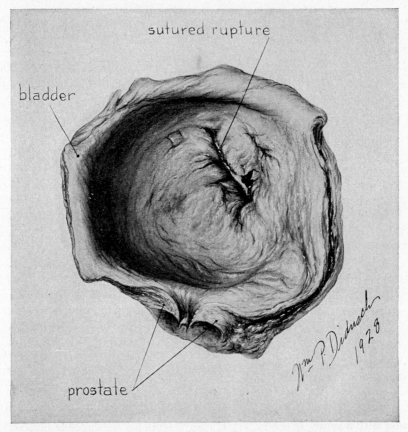

Fig. 16.—Rupture of a tabetic bladder (from the collection of the late Dr. F. Christeller, Virchow's Krankenhaus, Berlin; Lowsley and Kirwin: Clinical Urology. Williams and Wilkins Co.).

ally more severe, and, in addition, there are likely to be symptoms of peritonitis, unless the patient is seen early.

Intraperitoneal Rupture.—The common *early symptoms* are shock, which may be slight or so severe as to cause death; pain and tenderness in the hypogastrium, and a marked desire to void, with inability to do so or, at most, the passage of a few drops of blood. Occasionally there may be ability to void immediately after the accident, but evacuation will be painful and urine bloodstained. The abdominal distention, rigidity, and tenderness increase with the extravasation of urine, but gastro-intestinal symptoms are usually absent until peritonitis develops. If the urine is infected at the time of injury, the *later symptoms* are those of a septic peritonitis.

Extraperitoneal Rupture.—Early symptoms may be few or entirely lacking. If incurred in association with fracture of the pelvis, the symptoms produced by the fracture may temporarily mask the manifestations of the vesical injury, and it is only when the extravasated urine has had time to burrow into the surrounding tissues that the gravity of the vesical injuries is manifested. With *subsequent infection,* the clinical picture becomes that of sepsis. The pain following extraperitoneal rupture may be localized in the suprapubic region or referred to the perineum, rectum, penis, or lower extremities. There may be the passage of bloodstained urine or total inability to void. If the site of the rupture is in the base of the bladder, the urine usually will extravasate first into the most dependent part of the extravesical space; that is, the region occupied by the seminal vesicles behind the prostate, and, even if the rupture is higher up, the fluid will later invade this area. Its course may be upward, behind the posterior parietal peritoneum, in which case a mass may be palpated above the iliac crest or in one or both loins. In some instances there has even been invasion of the thigh, the extravasating urine dissecting under Poupart's ligament, generally external to the internal iliac vessels; or it may reach the scrotum, along and external to the structures occupying the inguinal canal. Extravasations can penetrate the pelvic fascia into the ischiorectal space and perineum, but this is unlikely unless the trauma causing the rent in the bladder has also caused disruption of other structures which normally would act as natural barriers.

Diagnosis (see also p. 142)

Intraperitoneal rupture, in particular, frequently takes place without any associated injuries.

The *history* and *physical examination* are important. A history of injury to the lower part of the abdomen, followed by hypogastric pain and intense desire to void with inability to do so, or by the passage of bloody urine, should arouse suspicion of rupture of the bladder. The presumptive diagnosis of rupture is strengthened by the presence of a palpable mass in the lower part of the abdomen or in the retrovesical region, or by free fluid in the abdomen, but these are later manifestations and to wait for their appearance is likely to prove disastrous.

When vesical injury is suspected, the patient should be requested to empty the bladder. His ability to pass urine which is not macroscopically bloody will be a fairly reliable indication that the bladder is intact.

Procedures.—The most commonly employed diagnostic procedure has been catheterization. Its use confirms an empty bladder or the presence of a small amount of bloody urine. Another method is to *instil a measured quantity* of sterile fluid and immediately attempt to withdraw it. If the amount recovered is less than that introduced, rupture should be suspected. *Cystoscopy* is sometimes useful in demonstrating the presence and location of small ruptures, but with larger tears, the inability to keep the bladder sufficiently distended and the excessive bleeding may make determination of the injury impossible. In many cases the associated injuries and the patient's general condition make cystoscopy entirely out of the question. *Injection cystography* and *aerograms* are also of value in demonstrating injury. However, neither a catheter nor a cystoscope can be used without risk of additional traumatization and increase in the incidence of infection. When the necessary time for the procedure can be allowed, diagnosis is best made by *intravenous urography,* which permits secretory cystograms showing the diffused dye outside the bladder. This procedure lessens the danger of infection. Because of the frequency of associated injury to the bladder, in all cases of fractured pelvis early intravenous urographic study should be made unless the patient can pass normal quantities of urine.

Immediate *exploratory operation,* preceded by transfusion, if necessary, is advisable in all cases in which the diagnosis is in doubt but the history and findings indicate rupture. Rupture of the bladder, particularly the intraperitoneal variety, requires emergency surgical procedures, and a favorable outcome is dependent on the length of time that elapses between receipt of the injury and institution of efficient drainage.

Prognosis

The prognosis, particularly in *intraperitoneal rupture,* is grave. The primary shock and hemorrhage may be so severe as to be rapidly fatal, or death may occur from peritonitis, rapid sepsis due to early infection developing in the extravasated tissues, or from associated injuries. *Early recognition and correction are of primary importance.* The high mortality in intraperitoneal ruptures has been due largely to failure to recognize the condition early enough for operation to be performed before infection has set in. *Extraperitoneal ruptures,* if uncomplicated, are usually less dangerous. An increasing proportion of these cases, however, are associated with fracture of the pelvis and extensive injury to adjacent structures.

The mortality of rupture of the bladder is necessarily dependent in part on the extent of general injuries, but it can be materially reduced by early diagnosis and operation.

Treatment

The treatment consists of supportive measures (such as transfusions, heat, and stimulants) and emergency surgical procedures.

OPERATIVE TREATMENT

Anesthesia

Operations on the bladder are frequently done under *regional* or *local* anesthesia. Local infiltration anesthesia, with *procaine,* 1 per cent, may be used if cystostomy only is to be performed (Fig. 17). Of late, spinal anesthesia has been used in the great majority of operations on the bladder.

For children and highly nervous patients, general inhalation anesthesia is preferable.

Preoperative Preparation

The preoperative preparation of the patient is most important. Usually, if the bladder shows signs of infection, vesical irrigations with suitable antiseptic solutions are given for several days before operation, and urinary antiseptics are given orally, but in emergencies these preliminaries sometimes must be dispensed with. Fluids should be taken freely up to the time of operation, unless inhalation anesthesia is to be used.

The patient is prepared in the customary manner in regard to catharsis and enemas. A soapsuds enema is given the evening before the operation, and a sedative, such as *phenobarbital* or *pentobarbital sodium,* 1½ grains (0.1 gm.), to insure a restful night. If regional anesthesia is to be used, the patient is permitted a light breakfast and fluids.

One hour before being sent to the operating table he is given additional analgesic medication by mouth. *Phenobarbital* or *pentobarbital sodium,* 3 grains (0.2 gm.), is satisfactory.

The skin of the abdomen and pubes is shaved and cleansed with tincture of green soap and warm water, followed by alcohol, 70 per

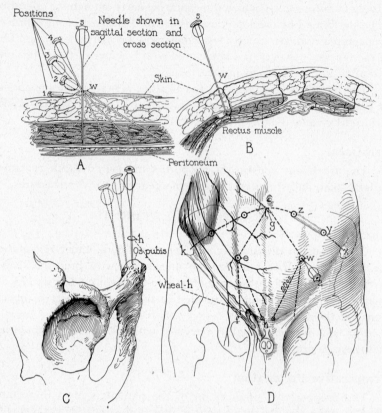

Fig. 17.—Abdominal block. The injection consists of 100 cc. of 0.5 per cent procaine solution at body temperature with 6 minims of 1:1000 epinephrine (1 cc. ampule, 1:2600). Anesthesia is induced in ten minutes and lasts one hour. The three zones of injection are shown in D. In order of the frequency of use they are: e to f and e to g (no hernia present); e to h and e to g (reducible hernia present); k to g (irreducible hernia present). All are bilateral. The blocks e to f, e to g, and e to h are made from wheal w, as shown in A, B, and D. The space of Retzius is injected from wheal h (C and D), 10 cc. on each side. Wheal w is shown in sagittal section in A, in cross-section in D and from in front in D. It is placed in the skin at the border of the rectus muscle midway between the umbilicus and pubes. In D the appearance of the skin is shown after a solution has been injected from y to z through the needle in A in first position. In B and D, the nerves to be blocked are shown in heavy black lines. In A the needle is shown in five positions in each of which 2 cc. of solution is used. Thus a 10 cc. syringe contains enough solution to block a brick-shaped area, a lateral view of which is shown in A. Such blocks, like bricks under various arrangements, result in the various types of abdominal block shown. In D, the lines ef, eg, and eh each traverses the ventral face of a brick-shaped block of anesthetized tissue. In the average case two injections of 10 cc. each are made into each brick; the second reinforces the first one (Lundy, J. S.: J. Urol., June, 1927).

cent, and sprayed with tincture of merthiolate (or other preferred antiseptic).

Just before the operation, a urethral catheter is introduced into the bladder, and the bladder is irrigated and moderately distended with

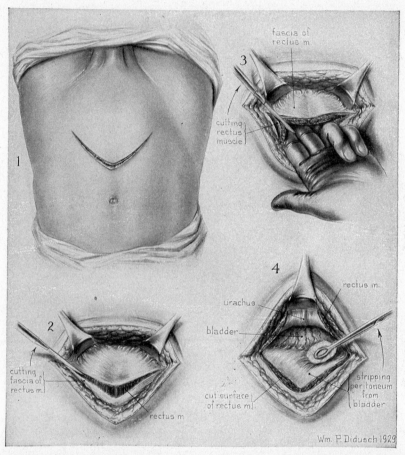

Fig. 18.—Suprapubic cystostomy. *1,* Inverted-V incision through the skin. *2,* The incision is deepened through the fascia of the rectus muscle on each side. *3,* The rectus muscle may be cut through, as illustrated here, or separated and retracted. *4,* Dissection is carried down along the urachus until the top of the bladder is reached; the peritoneum is then carefully pushed back, exposing the vault of the bladder (Lowsley and Kirwin: Clinical Urology. Williams and Wilkins Co.).

acriflavine, 1:6000, the end of the catheter being clamped to prevent outflow of the fluid. The patient is placed on the operating table in the Trendelenburg position.

Incisions for Approaching Bladder

There are a number of incisions for approaching the urinary bladder. The *vertical incision in the midline* is the one most commonly used. Some surgeons prefer the transverse incision. The *Pfannenstiel*

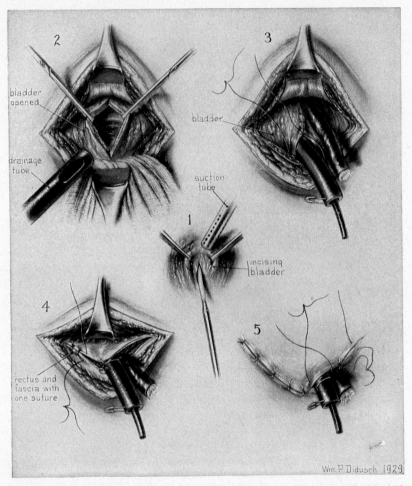

Fig. 19.—Suprapubic cystostomy. *1,* The bladder wall is grasped with Allis clamps, incised, and the bladder drained of fluid by a suction tube. *2* and *3,* If a plain cystostomy is being done, a Kenyon double suction tube is fixed at the highest point of the bladder incision by a catgut suture tied around it and sutured at the apex of the V. A cigarette drain is inserted over the suture line. *4,* The layers of muscle and fascia are repaired with plain catgut. *5,* The skin is sutured with silkworm gut, and the double suction tube fixed with one suture. By fixing the tube at the bladder and skin, the dead space is eliminated and the tube is brought through the abdominal wall obliquely (Lowsley and Kirwin: Clinical Urology. Williams and Wilkins Co.).

curved incision is often considered desirable when wide resection of the bladder, for tumor or diverticulum, is to be done.

In operations on the bladder, a large number of surgeons prefer the *inverted-V incision* (Figs. 18, 19). The apex of this should be well above the point to which the dome of the distended bladder would reach. For an ordinary suprapubic cystostomy, the incision is made so that the apex of the inverted V comes at a point about three-fourths of the distance between the symphysis pubis and the umbilicus. In cases in which wider exposure of the bladder is required, such as resection of the bladder for vesical neoplasm with transplantation of a ureter, or resection of a vesical diverticulum, the incision of choice is the Pfannenstiel, which lays open the entire pelvis.

Surgical Treatment of Rupture and Wounds of Bladder

Rupture of the bladder is an *emergency condition* of the first magnitude. The diagnosis should be made and surgical treatment instituted within a few hours. Negley in 1937 showed that the mortality rate for operations performed in the first twelve hours was only 11 per cent; in the second twelve hours, 22 per cent; and on the second day, 43 per cent. When the history and findings indicate rupture or a penetrating wound of the bladder, even if the diagnosis has not been definitely established, suprapubic exploration of the bladder is advisable, since delay in treatment is fatal.

The procedure to be followed will vary with the location of the rupture, the presence or absence of infection, and the associated injuries. In general, the *primary aims* of the surgical procedure are the repair of the rent, drainage of the infiltrated tissues, and drainage of the bladder.

Suprapubic Drainage.—The establishing of free suprapubic drainage, at the earliest moment, is of the utmost importance in all cases of rupture of the bladder, whether the rupture be extraperitoneal or intraperitoneal. In small, uncomplicated extraperitoneal ruptures and wounds, adequate suprapubic drainage of the bladder may be all that is necessary, if extravasation has not yet set in. In most instances, however, extravasation has already taken place, and abdominal, prevesical, and even perineal drainage may be needed in addition to cystostomy.

Intraperitoneal Rupture.—If intraperitoneal rupture is present, the fluid is aspirated. The vesical tear is located and repaired with catgut, and the peritoneum closed, if the patient is seen early, before infection has set in. Suprapubic drainage of the bladder, with a double suction tube, keeps the viscus dry and prevents urinary leakage, and should be maintained until healing takes place. If there has been extravasation of urine into the peritoneal cavity, a drain is placed in the cavity. Flushing out the abdominal cavity in cases of intraperitoneal rupture is considered unnecessary by most authors.

In very extensive lacerations of the bladder and adjacent tissues, the precarious condition of the patient may make complete repair inadvisable. In such cases it is wiser to control hemorrhage, provide free drainage, and administer supportive treatment.

Extraperitoneal Rupture.—In extraperitoneal rupture the rent usually occurs just behind the interureteral ridge, where it is easily identified and closed with two or three plain catgut sutures. The bladder is then closed around a double suction tube, and the skin incision closed in the usual manner.

Floor of Bladder.—Injuries involving the floor of the bladder, which have resulted in extravasation of urine deep into the pelvis, may require perineal as well as suprapubic drainage.

Rupture at Vesical Neck.—Of late years another type of extraperitoneal rupture has occasionally occurred, namely, rupture at the vesical neck, caused by the electrical loop used in the vesical-neck resection. When this occurs, in spite of the fact that the patient is under spinal anesthesia, he will complain bitterly of pain as the fluid passes out into the perivesical tissues. The course of procedure in such instances is immediate suprapubic cystostomy, with drainage both inside and outside the bladder, the tear being stitched up if it can be located (and it usually can be).

CHAPTER IV

CARE OF THE NEUROGENIC BLADDER

FRANK HINMAN, M.D.

THE care of the paralytic bladder is a grave responsibility. In the war of 1914–1918 about eight of every ten American and English soldiers sustaining injuries of the spinal cord which gave rise to a paralytic bladder died from this cause rather than from the injury. Death was caused by renal sepsis and decubital ulcers, and the fundamental basis of the teaching of this text is to reduce these hazards to a minimum. Unfortunately in time of war paralyzed men occasionally must endure periods of neglect. A break in methodical care, no matter how short, usually means disaster. There can be no set rule of treatment. The method of choice must vary with circumstances. The authoritative views on the subject, however, approve the precepts and precautions that are to be listed next.

Precepts

1. Prefer *noncatheterization* and *manual expression* of urine to all other methods.
2. Use a *retention catheter* with *continuous tidal irrigation* when the first-mentioned method fails, cannot be employed, or is contra-indicated.
3. Perform *suprapubic cystostomy* and establish *continuous tube drainage* whenever indicated, either by failure of the foregoing methods or for some other reason. An uncared-for suprapubic tube is preferable to distention and overflow.

As important as the foregoing doctrine of choice in the method of treatment are medical foresight and nursing vigilance.

Precautions

1. Never under any circumstances choose the method of *distention* and *overflow*. This is nothing but neglect. When faced by its unavoidable occurrence follow the foregoing precepts.
2. Never employ *intermittent catheterization*. If a catheter must be used, leave it in.
3. Never let a paralyzed bladder become *overdistended*, whatever method is selected. In other words, manual expression requires constant vigilance and must be performed at regular intervals; tube drainage, whether by urethral or suprapubic catheter, must be continuous, never intermittent. The retained catheter, furthermore, must never be shut off.

187

Definition

Any vesical disturbance (retention, dribbling, incontinence) caused by a lesion in the nervous system constitutes a neurogenic bladder. The term "cord bladder" is applied to vesical dysfunction arising from a lesion in the spinal cord. In civil life, tabes dorsalis and the various other forms of syphilis of the central nervous system account for more than 80 per cent of all neurogenic bladders. The discussion in this chapter is not concerned with this type of "cord bladder."

Etiology

In military practice, the majority of neurogenic bladders result from *injuries to the spinal cord;* a few are observed as a complication of *injuries to the brain;* fewer still are caused by damage to the peripheral ganglia and nerves supplying the bladder. In contrast to civil practice very few will be caused by disease.

Trauma to the nervous system (brain, spinal cord, peripheral ganglia, and nerves) may be inflicted by the direct action of a penetrating missile, by displaced fragments of bone, or by hemorrhage. It may likewise occur through the medium of secondary infection. The formation of scar tissue and the growth of new bone late in the course of healing of various injuries mentioned may contribute additional damage.

A concussion is a mild, transient form of injury caused by pressure which is usually the result of edema. Compression or a partial division of nerve fibers is more serious. Such an injury may be followed by a more or less complete return of function; on the other hand, the initial disability may prove permanent. Complete destruction of nerve fibers, of course, precludes any possibility of repair (paralysis).

Physiology

Nerves in Bladder Mechanism.—Three sets of nerves supply the bladder and control micturition: (1) the sympathetic nerves (hypogastric from the lumbar segment of the spinal cord), (2) the parasympathetic nerves (pelvic from sacral segment), and (3) the somatic nerves (pudic from sacral segment).

Although knowledge concerning the autonomic *sympathetic* pathway (hypogastric) is incomplete, this set of nerves probably receives its connections from the spinal cord between the second thoracic and third lumbar segments, inclusive. Physiologically, the sympathetic nerves control mainly the involuntary mechanism of filling of the bladder. Their stimulation causes relaxation of the detrusor muscle and contraction of the internal urinary sphincter.

The autonomic *parasympathetic* nerves (pelvic) communicate with the spinal cord through the second and third sacral nerves. They control the involuntary mechanism of emptying of the bladder. Their stimulation produces contraction of the detrusor muscle and relaxation of the internal sphincter.

The *somatic* nerves (pudic) arise from the third and fourth sacral segments. They serve in the voluntary control of micturition and supply the external urinary sphincter, the adjacent portion of the urethra, and the accessory urethra and perineal muscles.

Nervous Centers.—Five nervous centers are concerned in the regulation of micturition: (1) the cerebral, (2) the subcortical, (3) the lumbar, (4) the sacral, and (5) the ganglionic in the peripheral plexuses.

All voluntary impulses arise in the cerebral center. The remaining centers are thrown into voluntary activity by impulses transmitted from this governing station or by reflexes originating in the peripheral nerves. Those pathways by which micturition is controlled are in the most dorsal part of the lateral column and in the region of the pyramidal tract. One such pathway on each side is sufficient to maintain control, provided the one on the other side is not impaired. There is much decussation of the fibers in both the lumbar and sacral centers.

Normally the impulse to urinate originates in the brain and is delivered by the midbrain to the spinal centers, exciting various nervous reflexes into automatic action. Through the hypogastric nerves flash inhibitory signals to the detrusor muscle and stimulating impulses to the sphincter; whereas, reciprocally antagonistic impulses flow through the pelvic nerves, stimulating the detrusor muscle and inhibiting the sphincter. These reflex impulses show an integrative activity not unlike peristalsis. The trigonal muscle has sympathetic innervation only, no parasympathetic, so that, with sympathetic inhibitory impulses to the detrusor muscle, stimulating impulses flow to the trigon. The striated muscles receive voluntary impulses through the pudendal nerve.

Sympathetic-Parasympathetic Balance.—The mutual antagonism of the sympathetic supervision of vesical filling and the parasympathetic supervision of vesical emptying is only partial. One does not become dominant with the loss of the other. An intact parasympathetic pathway is more essential, however, than an unbroken sympathetic one. A neurogenic disorder of the bladder occurs whenever a lesion in any of the centers of micturition, in any of their connecting pathways, or in any of their peripheral connections supplying the bladder and the urethra, disturbs that fine balance existing between the two mechanisms. An overactivity of the sympathetic nerves results in an atonic neurogenic bladder, and a spastic, hypertonic type of neurogenic bladder is observed when the parasympathetic nerves gain control. Mixed types of disorder likewise occur.

Pathology

The common effect on micturition of a transverse lesion at any level of the cord or cauda equina may be described in three phases. These are: (1) retention, (2) overflow incontinence, and (3) automatic micturition.

Urinary Retention.—The first or atonic phase is constant for all lesions, although variable in duration. In fractures below the lumbar center, the other effects may be slight or absent. The phase of urinary retention commonly lasts from two to three weeks but may disappear within twenty-four hours or persist for eighteen or more months. Retention, in the presence of injury at any level, is explained on the basis of "spinal shock" which isolates the bladder from its reflex centers. Complete paralysis of the detrusor muscle and spasm of the sphincter result. Because of this spasm, catheterization usually is difficult. Reflex contractility is entirely absent.

Overflow Incontinence.—The second phase should be prevented from occurring since it delays and compromises the development of an automatic bladder. As the bladder becomes more and more distended the intravesical pressure rises so high that, barring a mechanical obstruction, the urine is forced through the sphincters and dribbles from the urethra, and overflow incontinence exists. Occasionally this is the final phase after destructive lesions of the sacral segments or the cauda equina.

Automatic Micturition.—The third phase is the development of an automatic bladder. Occasionally recovery is complete and normal voluntary micturition is restored, but more commonly a spastic neurogenic bladder develops and periodic reflex micturition (the automatic bladder) is established as a permanent state. With the gradual gain in muscle tone, contractility slowly returns to the detrusor muscle, and subsequently it hypertrophies. Along with this recovery of the detrusor muscle there is return of sphincteric spasm so characteristic of the first phase. The insertion and retention of a catheter again become more difficult.

In fully developed reflex micturition the bladder functions purely as a reflex organ. When the set capacity has been reached, the detrusor muscle contracts, the sphincter relaxes, and the urine is discharged in a powerful stream. This is purely an involuntary act, and in most instances the patient is unaware that micturition is taking place. Automatic micturition occurs sooner and more perfectly after fractures above the lumbar center than after those below that point. It differs from normal micturition in the incoordination of detrusor muscle and sphincter. Instead of being reciprocal, their activity becomes synchronous. With the return of its tone and contractility, the detrusor muscle, in order to establish automaticity, must work against the unwonted coincidental contraction of the sphincter, and, with good automaticity, it will hypertrophy and the bladder will return to normal dimensions. So high may this initial return of tonus become sometimes that, unless preventive measures are instituted, the capacity of the bladder will be reduced to almost nothing. The smallest amounts of urine set up emptying contractions so that the patients are as incontinent as in the previous phase, but for another reason.

In the atonic phase all of the spinal reflexes below the level of the lesion are abolished. The return of the spinal reflexes announces the development of the spastic stage which is fully established when hyperreflexia and positive Babinski reflex are noted.

Occasionally there is recurrence of attacks of retention with temporary reversion to the atonic state after reflex micturition has been established. This is especially true of lesions of the cauda equina and during severe toxemia from infection.

In the extremes between hypertrophy and atony of the detrusor muscles, partial and atypical forms of an automatic bladder may be observed.

Symptoms

Urinary Retention.—The cardinal symptom of the *atonic neurogenic bladder* is urinary retention. When produced by spinal shock, the initial phase is complete retention, which gradually gives way to overflow of urine (passive incontinence). The capacity of the bladder is enormous, and vesical distention may prove exquisitely painful, while at other times the patient is entirely unaware that it exists. Hematuria is sometimes observed in the early stages of an atonic bladder of this type. The bleeding, which may prove alarming, is induced by vasomotor changes which occur in the bladder.

Urinary Incontinence.—In a *spastic neurogenic bladder* active urinary incontinence (periodic reflex micturition) is the rule. When the damage to the nerve is not very severe, however, the patient may exert a certain amount of voluntary control, when urinary frequency, urgency, and dysuria are complained of. The bladder is never so widely distended in the spastic disorder as in the atonic and rarely ever presents above the symphysis pubis.

Complications

Urinary Infection.—A death rate of 80 per cent from urinary infection during the war of 1914–1918 is overwhelming evidence of the appalling nature of this complication. Infection of the bladder is not in itself lethal, but it is a source of great potential danger in that it often leads to ascending infection and the development of pyelonephritis. It has been observed in this condition that urinary infection is almost invariably introduced by urethral instrumentation, such as the passage of a catheter. Fortunately it has become increasingly more evident that the danger of extension to the upper part of the urinary tract is directly proportional to the degree of vesical distention. When the cystitis is kept under control by proper methods of treatment, as will be outlined, and no obstruction or reflux from distention is allowed to occur, the incidence of pyelonephritis becomes negligible and, when it does occur, it is rarely fatal.

Local Effects of Inflammation.—A virulent cystitis has severe local effects even if it does not immediately lead to a fatal ascending infection. Early in the course of a spastic neurogenic bladder, cystitis causes such irritation that the capacity of the bladder is reduced to between 30 and 60 cc., with the result that the patient suffers from an almost continuous escape of urine. Subsequently there is destruction of the musculature of the wall of the bladder and replacement with scar tissue which may render this disability permanent.

Decubital Ulcers.—Another serious complication of spinal injuries is the development of decubital ulcers. These attain added virulence if soiled with urine, a danger which is ever imminent in urinary incontinence.

Obstructive Complications.—The retention of urine in the uninfected bladder does not give rise to the obstructive complications that might be anticipated. Rupture of the bladder is extremely rare, even in complete retention, provided no infection or mechanical obstruction exists. The intravesical pressure forces the sphincters, which allow the escape of urine before a rupture occurs. Hydronephrosis and renal insufficiency from back-pressure do not occur unless the changes incident to infection cause a narrowing of the lower end of the ureter.

Calculi.—A fairly common complication of prolonged cystitis is the deposition of calcareous deposits on the mucosa of the bladder.

Vesical calculi are likewise prone to occur, especially if the urine is alkaline.

Diagnosis

The diagnosis of a neurogenic bladder presents no difficulty in the presence of typical lesions of nerves, and the symptoms and neurologic signs yield sufficient evidence to classify properly the type, as previously discussed under the physiology and pathology of the condition. In practice, when the patient is seen soon after injury, the level of the injury has little significance. Vesical retention is the effect of injuries from the brain to the cauda equina, and management of the condition will differ in no essential points.

The cystoscope is rarely needed in making the diagnosis except to rule out a mechanical obstruction. Indeed, unless some special indication for its use is present, the passage of a cystoscope is just as undesirable as the introduction of a urethral catheter. This will be discussed under "Treatment."

Cystoscopy in Atonic Bladder.—The cystoscopic picture of an atonic neurogenic bladder is that of a widely dilated cavity; the vesical wall is pale and smooth. In cases of long duration fine trabeculations which result from muscular atrophy may be observed posterior to the ureteral orifices. The urethra and bladder are usually so insensitive that cystoscopy causes slight if any discomfort. The capacity of the bladder ranges from 500 to 1500 cc., with a general average of 1000 cc. The amount of residual urine usually present is 80 per cent of the total amount of urine that the bladder can hold. When infection occurs, inflammatory changes can be seen, and the capacity and amount of residual urine are markedly reduced.

Cystoscopy in Spastic Bladder.—In a spastic neurogenic bladder the capacity is small; it averages from 60 to 300 cc., and the amount of residual urine fills from 20 to 40 per cent of the bladder. In the presence of infection the capacity is rarely more than from 30 to 60 cc. Cystoscopy may be painful, and if fluid is introduced in excess of the vesical capacity it is discharged in a forceful stream around the cystoscope. Gigantic trabeculae from hypertrophy of the detrusor muscle completely fenestrate the interior of the bladder.

Differential Diagnosis.—Most important in the differential diagnosis is the elimination of the presence of a mechanical obstruction as the sole cause of the symptoms or as coexisting with a neurogenic bladder. Short of cystoscopy this may be done by obtaining a previous history of urinary difficulty, by palpating the urethra for the presence of a stricture, by examining the perineum, the external genitalia, and the pelvis for any sign of injury to eliminate the possibility of a ruptured urethra, and by performing a gentle rectal examination to detect any prostatic enlargement.

Treatment

Principles.—In the treatment of neurogenic bladder the prime objectives are the prevention of renal infection and decubital ulcers and the acceleration of automatic micturition and the return of vesical function.

The *prevention of renal infection* is the first consideration in the selection of a method of treatment. It is so important, in fact, that the rules governing the choice of method were given to introduce the subject of the care of the paralytic bladder. These precepts and precautions are explained in some detail, and later, in conclusion, will again be repeated. Thrice read they should not be forgotten.

Precepts
1. Prefer *noncatheterization* and *manual expression* of urine to all other methods.
2. Use a *retention catheter* with *continuous tidal irrigation* when the first-mentioned method fails, cannot be employed, or is contraindicated.
3. Perform *suprapubic cystostomy* and establish *continuous tube drainage* whenever indicated, either by failure of the foregoing methods or for some other reason.

Equally important with this doctrine of choice in the method of treatment are the medical foresight and nursing vigilance.

Precautions
1. Never under any circumstances choose the method of *distention* and *overflow*. This is nothing but neglect. When faced by its unavoidable occurrence follow the foregoing precepts.
2. Never employ *intermittent catheterization*. If a catheter must be used, leave it in.
3. Never let a paralyzed bladder become *overdistended*, whatever method is selected. In other words, manual expression requires constant vigilance, and tube drainage, whether by urethral or suprapubic catheter, must be continuous. Manual expression must be done at regular intervals; catheterization must never be intermittent. The retained catheter, furthermore, must never be shut off.

The fatal consequences of urinary infection have already been outlined. It is obvious that the most desirable type of treatment prevents the entrance of infection into the bladder. Should infection occur, the task becomes more difficult, yet with proper care vesical infection can be reduced to a minimum and its spread to the upper part of the urinary tract be forestalled.

In order to prevent ascending infection, as well as to accelerate either the *return of normal function* or the *development of automatic emptying*, the paralyzed bladder must never be allowed to become overdistended. Once the detrusor muscle has lost its tonicity, emptying by its own contractions becomes temporarily impossible, and return of function is long delayed. Likewise, from the viewpoint of functional return, it is essential that severe infection be prevented; for with destruction of the musculature of the wall of the bladder and replacement with fibrous tissue, contraction is impossible.

In the practical application of these principles the surgeon must first rapidly determine the following facts concerning a patient who comes under his care:

Status of Bladder.—He must ascertain the status of the neurogenic bladder after once making the diagnosis and ruling out a mechanical obstruction. It is important to know whether the bladder is of the atonic or spastic type and what degree of function is present. Information gained by inquiry as to how long previously the injury was sustained, whether or not urine is being passed, how much the bladder is distended, and by testing out the spinal reflexes and the Babinski reflex usually establishes the stage and type of dysfunction.

Presence of Infection.—Equally important, or even more so, the surgeon must immediately ascertain whether urinary infection exists. The presence of appreciable quantities of pus and bacteria in a *freshly* voided or expressed specimen of urine, provided there is no urethral discharge, may be considered as certain evidence of infection which may be only vesical. An elevation of temperature with tenderness over the kidney is presumptive evidence of pyelonephritis.

The only three methods worthy of consideration in the care of the paralytic bladder, as already given in the outline, are as follows:

I. *Noncatheterization and Manual Expression of Urine.*—This is the only method by which urinary infection can be avoided. It is the least time-consuming method and the best for the welfare of the patient unless some contraindication exists. It is applicable in those cases in which there is no urinary infection and in which no mechanical obstruction exists. As soon as a patient who meets these criteria comes under the physician's jurisdiction, place him on the following regimen:

SCHEDULE FOR MANUAL EXPRESSION.—The bladder is to be emptied as completely as possible every four hours* (at 2 A.M., 6 A.M.,

---

* In some cases every six hours will be sufficiently frequent, but clocklike regularity must always be maintained.

10 A.M., 2 P.M., 6 P.M., and 10 P.M.); any deviation from a rigid time schedule markedly impairs the efficiency of the treatment and may result in failure. At these appointed times the surgeon or some trained assistant enlists the patient's cooperation by instructing him to strain and exert as much intra-abdominal pressure as possible. At the same time the surgeon massages the bladder from above downward toward the symphysis with the palms or ulnar surfaces of his hands. The bladder should never be squeezed. If it has been allowed to become too distended, manual expression may cause intense pain which may be relieved by the administration of morphine. Having the patient lie on his side may facilitate the process. In the stage of reflex activity the excitation of a mass reflex by stroking the sole of the foot may provide additional aid.

Meticulous attention to these few details during the early days of atonicity will accelerate the contraction of the bladder and markedly hasten the development of automatic micturition and save the patient from endless catheter care. As the patient gradually develops more and more power to empty his bladder, there is less and less need for manual expression.

CONTRAINDICATION.—The advent of infection is the one real contraindication to the use of this method. The urine should be examined every day, for it is extremely dangerous to employ manual expression in the presence of infection. Not only is there a possibility of rupturing the bladder, whose walls have been weakened by infection, but the attending residual urine increases the virulence of infection and thus causes severe damage to the bladder. The greatest hazard, however, is the imminence of ascending pyelonephritis.

COLLECTION OF URINE.—In the application of this method great care must be taken to see that the urine does not soil the patient's skin. The most satisfactory method of collecting the urine is to place the penis in a large glass urinal. The glass is helpful to the attendants in ascertaining when it is necessary to empty the urinal, which should never become so full that the penis is immersed in the urine. By keeping the urinals clean, fresh specimens of urine are readily collected at daily intervals in order to detect the earliest appearance of pus and bacteria. These should be searched for, not only in the wet drop of the centrifuged urine, but in the stained specimen.

II. *Retention Catheter with Continuous Tidal Irrigation.*—This constitutes the next most desirable method of treatment. It should be instituted whenever urinary infection is present, or whenever such infection develops during the method of treatment just described. The insertion of a retention catheter with the institution of tidal irrigation is likewise indicated when for any other reason the method of manual expression is found unsatisfactory or impractical. Occasionally, bleeding from the bladder will be so severe that catheterization becomes necessary. In other cases vesical distention may be so extreme and so painful that all attempts at manual expression result in failure. This is especially likely to occur when the institution of treatment is too long delayed, or if too long a period is allowed to elapse between expressions of urine. Occasionally, soiling with urine may present such a problem as to require catheterization, as in irrational patients.

PROCEDURE.—In carrying out this method a Foley urethral catheter (ordinarily F. 22 in size with a 5-cc. bag) is introduced into the bladder with strict aseptic precautions. The bag, which will retain it in the bladder, is then filled with 5 cc. of sterile fluid, and the channel to the bag is tied off. The bladder is emptied and, following an irrigation with an isotonic solution of boric acid (1.5 per cent), tidal irrigation is set in operation, as shown in the accompanyng diagram (Fig. 20). A solution of *boric acid* is used for the irrigating medium, and in the atonic type of bladder the level of the irrigating chamber is set just a few centimeters above the level of the bladder. As reflex activity is recovered, this level is raised. Once each week the catheter is removed so that the urethra can be cleansed and rested. In the presence of urethral discharge, however, the catheter should be changed at least every third day. It is left out for a period of from four to six hours, and is reinserted after thorough urethral irrigation and aseptic precautions.

IRRIGATING SOLUTIONS.—Under certain conditions a solution other than boric acid will be found useful for irrigations. A 3 per cent solution of *sodium citrate* is helpful in the presence of bleeding since it prevents the formation of clots. A 0.25 per cent solution of *phosphoric acid* or a 1:500 solution of *acetic acid* is valuable in the presence of alkaline cystitis and in the prevention of calcareous deposits and the formation of calculi within the bladder.

TERMINATING TREATMENT.—When an automatic bladder is being finally established, the catheter is left out from six to eight hours or longer, and the patient voids before its reinsertion. The amount of residual urine is then determined. If it is 100 cc. or more, the catheter is left in place, but if the amount is less the catheter can be removed and the patient can be catheterized two or three times each day, and the interval lengthened as the amount of residual urine approaches 25 cc. or less and automatic emptying becomes firmly established.

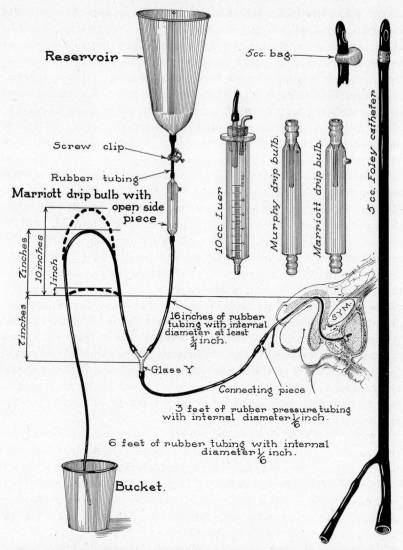

Fig. 20.—Apparatus for continuous tidal irrigation. Either a 10-cc. Luer syringe or a Murphy or Marriott drip bulb, as illustrated, may be used to provide a continuous drip. An air vent is essential in this unit. Sixty drops per minute is a suitable rate of flow from the antiseptic solution, as regulated by the screw clip. Since the solution is in contact with the vesical mucosa continuously a mild antiseptic, such as a 1.5 per cent solution of boric acid which is isotonic with the tissues, should be used. The height of the overflow tube above the symphysis pubis is adjusted according to the state of the neurogenic bladder. A height of about 2 inches is recommended for the atonic stage with gradual elevation to 10 inches or more as the hypertonic stage is reached. It is important to exclude all air in assembling the apparatus. This can be accomplished by con-

INTERMITTENT IRRIGATIONS.—During entrainment and under emergency conditions it is desirable to substitute intermittent irrigations temporarily for continuous tidal irrigation. Under these conditions the bladder must be irrigated twice daily with a quart of *boric acid* solution or 1:10,000 solution of *potassium permanganate*. Under no circumstances should the catheter be plugged between irrigations. It always should drain freely into a urinal or be connected with rubber tubing which remains open and drains into a gallon jug placed beneath the bed or stretcher.

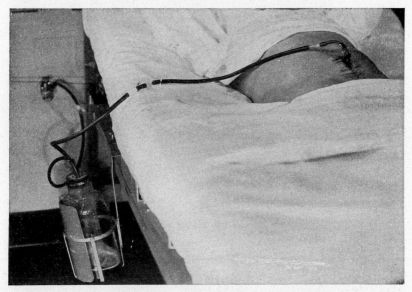

Fig. 21.—Suprapubic suction apparatus used at the Brady Foundation at the New York Hospital. The suction is furnished from a general system to a vacuum bottle held on the side of the bed by the angle frame. This is connected with the inner tube of a Kenyon double suction tube placed in the patient's bladder. Any fluid that arises in the outer tube is suctioned away by the inner tube (Lowsley and Kirwin: Clinical Urology. Williams and Wilkins Co.).

CARE OF CATHETER.—The care of a retention catheter is not simple. Tidal irrigations require constant supervision, and catheters

necting the rubber tubing to the catheter after the air bubbles have been evacuated from the tubing and while fluid is still running through the system and at the same time escaping from the bladder through the catheter. The reservoir must always contain fluid, and the end of the drainage tube must always be kept above the level of the fluid in the drainage bucket. As the bladder fills, the intravesical pressure rises until it reaches the level of the overflow tube, at which time siphonage takes place and the bladder empties. The cycle then starts again (after Lawrie-Nathan, 1939).

must be changed at regular intervals of from three to seven days. During certain phases (spastic) of vesical dysfunction, as mentioned previously, inlying catheters may be extruded or urine may leak around them. Such difficulties of insertion and retention complicate the problem of care.

III. *Suprapubic Cystostomy and Continuous Tube Drainage.*— This method is indicated for those patients of the preceding group who cannot tolerate a urethral catheter, for those who develop recurrent

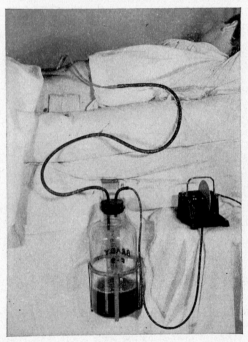

Fig. 22.—Stedman induction motor suction pump. Complete set-up, showing patient with double suction tube, collecting bottle, and Stedman suction pump in use. The dressings have been removed from the suprapubic wound (Lowsley and Kirwin: Clinical Urology. Williams and Wilkins Co.).

ascending infection on the regimen of urethral catheter drainage, for those who develop a virulent urethritis or an acute infection of the seminal tract such as an acute prostatitis or epididymitis, and for those who have vesical hemorrhage which is so severe that it cannot be controlled by a urethral catheter (Figs. 21, 22).

PROCEDURE.—The technic of suprapubic cystostomy should be simple and short. A long incision requiring sutures for closure is unnecessary when cystostomy is done for retention. There is no risk of peritoneal puncture when the bladder is distended. A large trocar and cannula can be safely plunged through a small slit in the skin, penetrating the bladder. After removal of the obturator, a bulb catheter (de Pezzer or Foley) of the appropriate size, previously stretched on a stylet, is passed into the bladder through the lumen of the cannula. The cannula is slipped out and the stylet removed. The catheter is pulled up gently until its mushroom end or bag impinges at the inner opening of the puncture wound in the dome of the bladder. Leakage of urine should not occur around the catheter. An anchor suture may be placed in the skin, and a small piece of gauze held by adhesive tape is the only dressing required.

The instructions regarding the care of a urethral catheter apply equally to the care of a suprapubic tube. Tidal irrigation is preferable to intermittent irrigations, provided there is no excessive leakage surrounding the tube.

When a spastic bladder has fully developed, the cystostomy tube is removed and a catheter inserted through the urethra. On healing of the suprapubic opening the urethral catheter is periodically removed in accordance with the instructions listed in the previous method.

CHEMOTHERAPY.—In addition to the purely local measures of treatment, urinary antiseptics may be administered by mouth. These will be found useful in the prevention as well as in the treatment of infections of the urinary tract. One of the preparations of mandelic acid, such as *elixir ammonium mandelate* in a daily dosage of 6 gm., divided into about four doses, constitutes one effective form of medication; the sulfonamide compounds, such as *sulfanilamide* or *sulfathiazole,* by mouth, 4 gm. daily, given in four divided doses for eight to ten days, are equally valuable. In many cases one of the sulfonamide compounds employed in the prevention or treatment of an infection of the spinal cord will exert a coincidental beneficial effect on the urinary tract.

Related Conditions

The activity of the *rectum* roughly parallels the sequence of events observed in the bladder. During the atonic stage there is marked relaxation of the entire rectum and of the anal sphincter, a helpful diagnostic sign. During this stage special attention must be paid to proper catharsis and the administration of daily enemas to assure proper elimination and to prevent fecal impactions.

Priapism may be one of the early manifestations of damage to the spinal cord. Later, erections are often caused by evoking the lower spinal reflexes. In the final stages of healing there is often persistence of a lack of sensation in the perineum and external genitalia, but at least a partial return of the sexual function is to be expected.

Prognosis

Only by preventing or controlling urinary sepsis can the appalling mortality incident to injuries of the spinal cord be reduced. In no other condition seen in military practice does the responsibility of the surgeon to prevent death and provide a good result assume such tremendous proportions. Aside from those cases in which normal micturition is restored, the best that can be anticipated is the establishment of an automatic bladder, but to accomplish either objective the patient must survive. Renal infection is the most frequent cause of death. With this uppermost in mind, the choice in the method of treatment must be made to fit conditions and circumstances.

Conclusions

Remember the three methods of treatment and their order of preference.

Precepts
1. Prefer *noncatheterization* and *manual expression* to all other methods.
2. Use a *retention catheter* with *continuous tidal irrigation* as the next method of choice.
3. Perform *suprapubic cystostomy* with *continuous tube drainage* whenever indicated.

Remember also the three important precautions.

---

1. Never under any circumstances choose the method of *distention* and *overflow*. This is nothing but neglect. When faced by its unavoidable occurrence follow the foregoing precepts.
2. Never employ *intermittent catheterization*. If a catheter must be used, leave it in.
3. Never let a paralyzed bladder become *overdistended* whatever method is selected. In other words, manual expression requires constant vigilance; and tube drainage, whether by urethral or suprapubic catheter, must be continuous, never intermittent. Expression must be done at regular intervals; catheterization must be continuous. The retained catheter, furthermore, must never be shut off.

CHAPTER V

INJURIES OF PENIS AND URETHRA, OF SCROTUM AND CONTENTS, AND OF PROSTATE GLAND AND SEMINAL VESICLES

HOMER G. HAMER, M.D.

THE PENIS

THESE injuries are infrequent and, when they occur, are likely to be associated with injuries to the urethra. However, severe injuries to the penis have occurred in cases in which the urethra was not involved. In civil practice, injuries to the penis include contusion, laceration, incision, puncture, denudation, dislocation, constriction, and the so-called "fracture." War wounds of the penis and urethra occur as the result of lacerations from high explosives and shrapnel as well as from gunshot wounds. Young and Davis reported forty-three cases of injury to the penile urethra or penis alone in the American Expeditionary Force (in the war of 1914–1918) in which the penis and urethra were injured. The penis may be completely severed, or the destruction may be so extensive that amputation is necessary.

Treatment

Simple *contusions* require only rest, elevation of the parts, and hot antiseptic applications (Fig. 23). *Subcutaneous hematoma* may necessitate incision and ligation of any bleeding vessels. Indications of *suppuration* or *emphysema* require immediate free incision and thorough drainage. If the *urethra* is involved, indwelling catheter drainage should be maintained until healing occurs. Should the injury be so extensive as to make catheterization impossible, perineal section or suprapubic cystostomy and retrograde catheterization may be required.

Incised wounds, if superficial, usually heal promptly. *Deep wounds* involving erectile tissue may cause severe hemorrhage. *Severance* of the penis may result fatally unless hemorrhage is promptly checked. *Arterial hemorrhage* should be controlled by ligation. *Venous oozing* ordinarily requires only coaptation of cut curfaces and compression, possibly aided by bandaging the penis, with a catheter in the urethra. *Puncture wounds* should be enlarged by incision to establish drainage and prevent infection. In *fracture* of the penis, clots may need to be evacuated and bleeding vessels ligated. Otherwise, compresses moistened in hot antiseptic solution or solutions of lead and opium may be all that is required. *Constriction* of the penis is usually promptly relieved by removal of the constricting band. If the

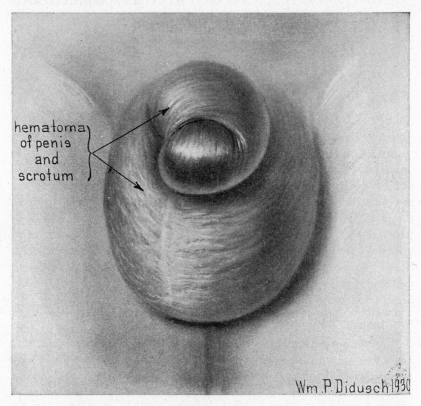

Fig. 23.—Hematoma of the penis and scrotum caused by slight contusion (Lowsley and Kirwin: Clinical Urology. Williams and Wilkins Co.).

latter is of metal, some ingenuity on the part of the surgeon may be required. Bandaging the organ tightly from before backward may reduce the edema sufficiently to allow the ring to be slipped off. If unsuccessful, metal-cutting tools may have to be employed.

THE URETHRA

The urethra may be punctured, incised, lacerated, or contused, or there may be a subcutaneous rupture. These injuries may be produced from within or from without.

INTERNAL INJURIES

Simple internal injury may be due to passage of foreign bodies or improper introduction of instruments. The bulb is most frequently traumatized from within. In stricture of the urethra, or hypertrophy of the prostate gland, the use of a urethrotome, lithotrite, or sound may cause injury with false passage.

The *symptoms* will depend on the extent of the injury. There may be only hemorrhage and painful urination. If the trauma is severe, there may be difficulty of urination, inflammatory swelling of the injured region with abscess formation, or extravasation of blood and urine.

EXTERNAL INJURIES

These include stab wounds, blows, falls, or crushing injuries with or without fracture of the pelvis. Injuries of the *pendulous urethra* are not very common, but may be caused by knife or gunshot wounds and have been observed as a result of violent coitus or breaking of a chordee.[9] Records of the American Expeditionary Force in the war of 1914–1918 include forty-three cases of injury of the penile urethra and ten of the deep urethra. In the *perineum* there is an additional cause, the straddle injury in which the urethra is crushed between the object and the pubes. The *membranous urethra* is most frequently injured indirectly as the result of fracture of the pelvis; a displaced fragment or splinter of the bone may lacerate the canal. The *prostatic urethra* is seldom injured from without except in fracture of the pelvis.

Pathology

Longitudinal incised wounds of the urethra heal readily with slight tendency to narrowing. If the injury is transverse, there is retraction of the segments, urine escapes, fibrous tissue forms between the segments, and stricture and urinary fistula result above the injury. In rupture of the *membranous urethra* from fracture of the pelvis and other causes, the urine and blood may collect in the pelvic tissue about the rectum, in the prevesical space, beneath the peritoneum or under the deep layer of the superficial fascia; the communication between the different layers of the tissues will depend on which layer of the urogenital diaphragm is lacerated. If the rupture involves the *perineal or pendulous portion* of the urethra, the extravasation of blood and urine may extend throughout the perineum, the scrotum, and the penis.

Symptoms (see also pp. 144, 145)

The symptoms of urethral injury due to external causes are pain, hemorrhage, disturbance of urination often involving retention and tumefaction. The development of these symptoms varies with the extent of the injury. There may be ecchymosis and swelling at the site

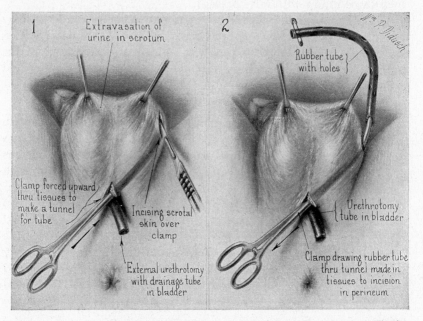

Fig. 24.—Extravasation of urine. Drainage of the scrotum (Lowsley and Kirwin: Clinical Urology. Williams and Wilkins Co.)

of the injury. In the severe cases hemorrhage is serious. Blood may appear at the meatus, flow back into the bladder or infiltrate the surrounding tissues. Efforts to urinate aggravate the pain and increase the swelling in the perineum. Diffuse extravasation of blood and urine rapidly develops (Figs. 24, 25). Chills and fever are almost invariably present. If operation is delayed, gangrene develops and sepsis is profound. The scrotum often sloughs away leaving the testes bare; perineal slough may also occur.

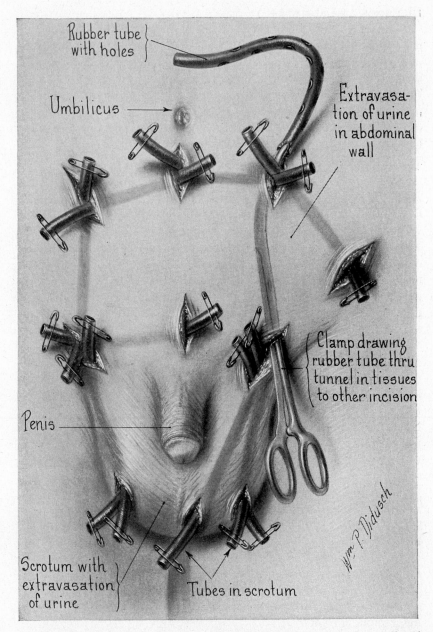

Fig. 25.—Extravasation of urine. Multiple incisions in abdominal wall and scrotum for free drainage of the extravasated region. The rubber tubes are drawn from one incision to another by a clamp (Lowsley and Kirwin: Clinical Urology. Williams and Wilkins Co.).

Diagnosis (see also p. 145)

Important points in diagnosis are the history and character of the injury, hemorrhage from the meatus and rapid development of perineal tumor. Retention usually signifies extensive injury. The diagnosis is more difficult in cases of fracture of the pelvis. Blood at the meatus may be absent. Retention of urine is almost invariably present. If crepitus is detected, roentgenography will demonstrate the fracture of the pelvis, and ineffectual efforts to catheterize would point to rupture of the membranous urethra.

Treatment

For simple injury, expectant treatment should be employed, including rest in bed, hot applications of antiseptic agents, urinary antiseptic agents administered internally, and irrigations of the urethra with *potassium permanganate* in 1:6000 or *silver nitrate* in 1:10,000 solution gently administered. Punctured wounds may require only compresses moistened in hot antiseptic solutions. If the urine is sterile and easily voided, no intra-urethral treatment is required. Severe injuries of the urethra, particularly perineal rupture, demand immediate perineal section for drainage and repair of the urethral wound (Figs. 26, 27). If the urethra is completely severed the proximal segment may be found with difficulty; often to accomplish this suprapubic cystostomy and retrograde catheterization are required. The divided ends of the urethra are united by interrupted catgut sutures, penetrating only the submucous layer. Attempt to unite the roof first. A catheter is then passed from the meatus into the bladder, the urethral gap closed, and drainage maintained through the suprapubic opening. Closure of the perineal wound, whether partial or complete, will depend on the presence or absence of infection. If damage to the urethral tissue is too great to permit suture, a perineal tube should be used for a few days and then followed by catheter drainage until healing is complete.

After-Treatment.—Urethral injuries, including contusions, are likely to be followed by stricture. Such strictures are prone to develop early, and often are resistant to treatment. In the milder injuries a full-sized sound should be used a few times and the patient warned of the danger of stricture. In severe cases sounds should be used once or twice a week for some weeks, and afterward at longer intervals, for months or years.

Prognosis

The dangers from rupture of the urethra are fatal hemorrhage, retention of urine, and uremia and sepsis attributable to urinary ex-

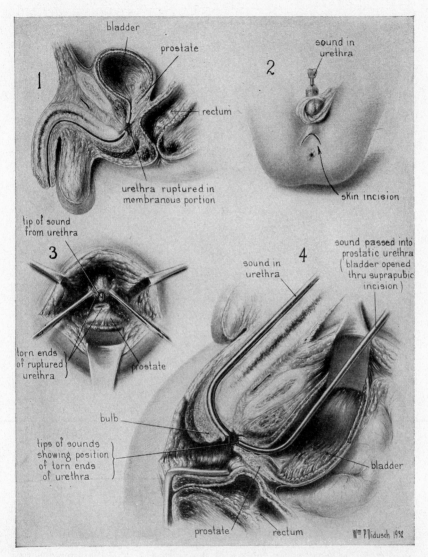

Fig. 26.—Operation for rupture of the urethra. *1,* Sagittal view, showing the urethra ruptured in the membranous portion. *2,* A sound is passed down to the rupture and an inverted-V incision made in the perineum and deepened to expose the membranous urethra. *3,* The tip of the sound can be seen in the severed distal end of the urethra. *4,* Sagittal view, illustrating the technic used when the lumen of the proximal end cannot be located. A suprapubic incision is made, and a sound passed through the vesical orifice and prostatic urethra, showing the location of the proximal end of the urethra (Lowsley and Kirwin: Clinical Urology. Williams and Wilkins Co.).

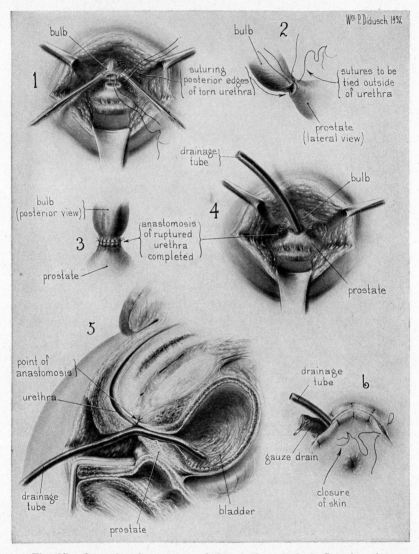

Fig. 27.—Operation for rupture of the urethra. *1, 2, 3,* Suturing the torn ends of the urethra. Only the posterior edges are sutured. *4,* View through the perineal wound, showing the anastomosis completed. The anterior wall is not sutured. A rubber tube or catheter is inserted for drainage. *5,* Sagittal view of the completed anastomosis. *6,* Final skin closure (Lowsley and Kirwin: Clinical Urology. Williams and Wilkins Co.).

travasation. The outlook is much more favorable if the condition is recognized early and prompt treatment is instituted. Late dangers are due to formation of stricture with resulting changes in the bladder and kidneys. If the infiltration is absent, the prognosis is more favorable.

THE SCROTUM

The scrotum may sustain extensive injury with little or no damage to its contents. Lacerations, incised wounds, gunshot wounds, stab wounds, and wounds following attempts at emasculation are seen and in some instances may be accompanied by loss of scrotal content. The injury may be such that the scrotum and skin of the penis are torn away. Records of the American Expeditionary Force[9] in the war of 1914–1918 list 164 injuries to the scrotum, with 5 deaths from injury of the scrotum and 10 deaths from injury of the testicle.

Treatment

The injuries should be treated according to recognized surgical principles. When penetrating injuries are sustained, hemostasis must be accomplished immediately lest hematoma form. Apposition of the edges of the skin should be done carefully because of its tendency to inversion. The scrotum has remarkable power of regeneration even after extensive loss of tissue from trauma or gangrene. If the testicles are devoid of scrotal covering, regeneration will take place. Convalescence may be hastened by constructing a scrotum with skin flaps.

Prognosis

Physiologic and cosmetic results are good owing to the surprising ability of the scrotum to regenerate.

THE TESTICLES IN GENERAL

These injuries are relatively infrequent. The protection is greater than usually thought. Because of free mobility and their suspended position they move away from the lines of force of blow or penetrating injuries.

Wounds may be open or closed. *Open wounds* include punctured, lacerated stab, or gunshot injuries along with those wherein the scrotum and enveloping tunics have been torn or incised. *Closed wounds* may be in the form of contusions or dislocations or injury to the blood vessels of the spermatic cord. Laceration or severance of the vas deferens may occur. Closed wounds of the testicle are most frequently sustained when the victim falls astride some object or while riding horseback. Kicks are also commonly the cause of such injuries.

Symptoms

The immediate effect of these injuries is swelling and edema of the scrotum, ecchymosis, and pain extending from the testicles to the thighs and abdominal region. The testicle is enlarged and painful to

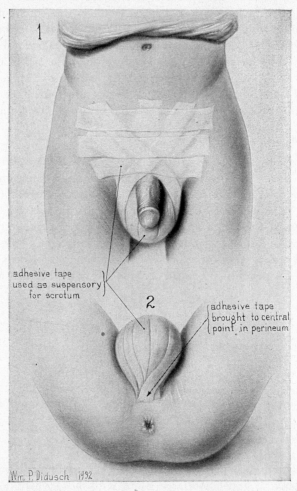

adhesive tape used as suspensory for scrotum

adhesive tape brought to central point in perineum

Wm. P. Didusch 1932

Fig. 28.—Adhesive tape suspensory for support of the scrotum in inflammatory conditions or following operation (Lowsley and Kirwin: Clinical Urology. Williams and Wilkins Co.).

palpation. The swelling and congestion increase for several hours, then begin to subside. Because of the inelasticity of the tunica albuginea, which limits swelling somewhat, pain may be intense and compression atrophy may result.

Treatment

Expectant or symptomatic treatment is usually all that is required, and this includes rest in bed, immobilization and elevation of the scrotum, application of ice bag, and analgesic agents (Fig. 28). Should a hematocele develop, early operation is indicated. Open the tunica vaginalis, remove the blood clots, and control the hemorrhage. The redundant tunica is trimmed away and the remainder everted as in operation for hydrocele. Orchidectomy may become imperative if the bleeding point cannot be found. If suppuration is evident, incise and drain.

LUXATION OF TESTICLE

Nearly always this is due to severe trauma wherein the scrotum is caught between the perineum, thigh or pubis and a foreign body.

Diagnosis

Swelling and discoloration of the scrotum develop early. If the patient is seen immediately after the injury, diagnosis can be made by the absence of the testicle from the scrotum. The testicle may be displaced in any one of many locations; for example, inguinal canal, shaft of penis, under the skin of the thigh, under the skin of the perineum, and above the pubic bone near the midline.

Treatment

This consists of replacement of the testicle in the scrotum, either by manipulation or by operative measures.

EPIDIDYMO-ORCHITIS OR TRAUMATIC EPIDIDYMITIS

Traumatic epididymitis existing as a clinical entity is highly problematical; the evidence is definitely against it. Because of the mobility of the testicle, injury sufficient to traumatize the epididymis is almost certain to injure the body of the testicle, hence the term "epididymo-orchitis" indicates the resulting pathologic condition.

Diagnosis

In the *rare cases* in which the epididymis alone is involved, there is definite swelling of the globus major and globus minor which is distinguishable from the testicle by palpation. In the *severe type* of epididymo-orchitis the entire half (if unilateral) of the scrotum may be filled by a firm, tender mass. In this instance little information is gained by palpation. Differentiation from infection is made by bacteriologic methods.

Treatment

Immobilization, together with elevation of the scrotum, is the keynote to the treatment. Ice bags help to relieve the pain; acetyl-salicylic acid in combination with an opiate may be necessary. If the swelling is not one of true epididymitis, but is due to hematoma, the treatment to be instituted is that recommended for hematocele.

THE VAS DEFERENS

These injuries may be due to ordinary trauma, stab wounds, bullet wounds, or lacerations; or to accidental operative injury or injuries attributable to antiseptic agents injected into its lumen.

Pathology

Any injury to the vas deferens is likely to result in occlusion. Trauma will probably result in greater injury to the blood vessels of the cord than to the vas itself.

Treatment

Traumatic injuries, lacerations, punctures, and contusions should be treated as wounds elsewhere. The primary point in repair of the vas is coaptation of the severed ends of the sheath. If this is done, regeneration can be expected.

THE PROSTATE GLAND AND SEMINAL VESICLES

These injuries seldom occur except as a part of injuries to the *pelvic bone,* particularly of the crushing type. Injuries of the prostate gland are usually associated with rupture of the bladder or of the deep urethra; these associated injuries demand attention more partic-ularly than the injury to the prostate. Injuries of the seminal vesicles are extremely rare even in connection with fracture of the bony pelvis. Like injuries to the prostate gland, they are seldom recog-nized and cause no symptoms in themselves. Penetrating wounds of the *rectum* in accidental injuries may also injure the prostate gland and seminal vesicles.

REFERENCES

1. Boyd, M. L.: Gunshot Wounds of the Bladder. J.A.M.A. *89:* 196–197 (July 16), 1927.
2. Cunningham, J. H., Jr.: Injuries and Infections of the Prostate and Seminal Vesicles. In Lewis, Dean: Practice of Surgery. Hagerstown, Maryland, W. F. Prior Company, Inc., 1940, Vol. 9, Chap. 18, pp. 1–24.
3. Eisendrath, D. N., and Rolnick, H. C.: Text-book of Urology. For Students and Practitioners. Philadelphia, J. B. Lippincott Company, 1928.

4. Hamer, H. G.: Anatomy, Malformations and Injuries of the Urethra. In Lewis, Dean: Practice of Surgery. Hagerstown, Maryland, W. F. Prior Company, Inc., 1940, Vol. 9, Chap. 22, pp. 1–28.
5. Hinman, Frank: The Principles and Practice of Urology. Philadelphia, W. B. Saunders Company, 1935.
6. Jeck, H. S.: Injuries of the Testis, Epididymis and Vas Deferens. Cyclopedia of Medicine, Surgery and Specialties. Philadelphia, F. A. Davis Company, 1940, Vol. 14.
7. Keyes, E. L.: Textbook on Urology. New York, D. Appleton and Company, 1928, 5th ed.
8. Lowsley, O. S., and Kirwin, T. J.: A Text-book of Urology. Philadelphia, Lea and Febiger, 1926.
9. Young, H. H., and Davis, D. M.: Young's Practice of Urology. Based on a Study of 12,500 Cases. Philadelphia, W. B. Saunders Company, 1926, Vols. 1 and 2.

CHAPTER VI

DO'S AND DON'T'S

FRANK HINMAN, M.D., CLARK M. JOHNSON, M.D., AND
H. M. WEYRAUCH, M.D.

THE KIDNEY: NONTRAUMATIC

DO

1. Obtain an uncontaminated specimen of urine either by catheterization or by the three-glass test, using the second glass for complete examination.

2. Ascertain the total renal function by a phthalein test.

3. Obtain a simple roentgenogram of the kidneys, ureters, and bladder in all cases of suspected urolithiasis; look it over carefully for stones in the region of the kidney or ureter, and note the size and position of the kidneys and the presence or absence of the psoas shadow on both sides.

4. Institute proper medical treatment in acute renal infection, either unilateral or bilateral, with urinary antiseptics and fluids for a reasonable length of time before going ahead with ureteral catheterization.

DON'T

1. Don't ever perform nephrectomy for any reason without ascertaining the presence of an adequate kidney on the opposite side.

2. Except in grave emergencies don't attempt cystoscopic examination to investigate infections of upper part of tract in the presence of virulent infection of the lower part of tract.

3. Don't make retrograde pyelograms on acutely infected kidneys except when absolutely necessary to make the diagnosis.

4. Don't subject infected kidneys to rough and repeated manual examination.

<table>
<tr><td>DO</td><td>DON'T</td></tr>
</table>

5. Eliminate all other possible causes as rapidly as possible in the presence of sepsis before subjecting the patient to cystoscopic examination.

6. Catheterize the ureter immediately when a pelvic stone seems to be blocking the ureter.

7. Leave ureteral catheters in place for drainage in unilateral or bilateral renal infection, when obstruction is present, as demonstrated at cystoscopic examination.

8. Obtain intravenous urograms whenever in doubt, and especially in the presence of marked infection when instrumentation might be harmful.

9. Remember that renal infection — pyelonephritis — is seldom fatal unless there is an obstruction in the urinary tract.

THE KIDNEY: TRAUMATIC

1. Obtain immediately intravenous urograms or retrograde pyelograms in all cases of suspected renal injuries.

2. Delay surgical intervention until the period of shock is over unless it is definitely apparent that massive renal hemorrhage is occurring as in cases of intraperitoneal rupture.

1. Don't hesitate to obtain retrograde pyelograms in cases of suspected renal injuries.

2. Don't neglect to look at the urine of every injured patient.

3. Don't attempt to do intravenous urograms on a patient in shock, or who has a temporary anuria.

DO

3. Obtain a specimen of urine at once from all patients who have sustained injury or gunshot wounds.

4. Obtain a catheterized specimen of urine, if the patient is unable to void and if it is befitting.

5. Investigate hematuria in each case, for it is a sign of injury somewhere along the urinary tract.

6. Treat renal injuries conservatively, except gunshot wounds, for the best results except in the presence of an increasing hematoma in the flank or continued profuse hematuria.

7. Institute surgical intervention for the injured kidney soon enough so that conservative methods of suturing may be instituted without endangering the patient's life.

8. Perform nephrectomy almost always for gunshot wound involving one kidney.

9. Investigate other visceral injuries which almost always accompany gunshot wound involving the kidney.

10. Investigate the kidney at the time of operation in all cases of abdominal gunshot wounds in which there is also hematuria.

11. Obtain half-hourly or hourly blood pressure and pulse readings on every patient who has a renal injury.

DON'T

4. Don't allow patients who have had an injury to the kidney, no matter how mild, out of bed in less than ten days.

5. Don't discharge patients who have had renal injuries until a check-up and cystoscopic examination are done to determine the remaining renal function and the pyelographic appearance of the kidney for future record.

DO　　　　　　　　　　　　**DON'T**

12. Get blood grouping on every patient suspected of having renal injuries.

THE URETER

1. Obtain a simple roentgenogram of the kidneys, ureters, and bladder in all cases of suspected ureteral stone.
2. Examine carefully the urine of all patients with ureteral colic for the presence or absence of blood and pus.
3. Pass ureteral catheters on all patients with proved or suspected renal stone, if there is anuria, and in all cases of ureteral injury, whether due to rupture by stone, abdominal operation, or by gunshot wound; apply adequate drainage extraperitoneally for the extravasated urine as an emergency measure.
4. Repair tears in ureters as soon as possible; in case of complete severance of the ureter by bullet, nephrectomy is usually indicated. See "Don't."

1. Don't ever attempt repair of a completely severed ureter without providing for urinary drainage above the site of the lesion.

THE BLADDER IN GENERAL

1. Suspect all patients who have had injury of having a ruptured bladder, especially those who have pelvic fractures.

1. Don't drain the peritoneum in intraperitoneal rupture of the bladder. Suture of the opening and suprapubic cystotomy only are indicated.

DO

2. Examine all injured patients for suprapubic tenderness, which is the cardinal point in vesical rupture.

3. When in doubt, catheterize patients who are suspected of having vesical rupture and make a cystogram after distending the bladder to its capacity with sodium iodide or some other radiopaque substance. Take a roentgenogram, allow the substance to flow out of the catheter, and take another.

4. Treat as emergencies all patients with bladders ruptured either by intravesical or extravesical force. Remember that all patients with intravesical ruptures should be operated on at once. The mortality rate after twenty-four hours is more than 50 per cent.

5. Perform cystotomy in cases of massive vesical hemorrhage in which the clots cannot be evacuated by suction with an instrument passed through the urethra.

6. Pass a catheter immediately into any bladder distended because of obstruction.

DON'T

2. Don't expect a rupture of the bladder, either intraperitoneal or extraperitoneal, to heal without surgical intervention.

3. Don't fail to provide adequate perivesical drainage in cases of extraperitoneal rupture.

THE NEUROGENIC BLADDER

1. Prefer noncatheterization and manual expression to all other methods.

2. Use a retention catheter with continuous tidal irrigation as the next method of choice.

1. Never under any circumstances choose the method of distention and overflow. This is nothing but neglect. (When faced by its unavoidable occurrence follow the precepts in the opposite column.)

DO

3. Perform suprapubic cystostomy with continuous tube drainage whenever indicated.

DON'T

2. Never employ intermittent catheterization. (If a catheter must be used, leave it in.)

3. Never let a paralyzed bladder become overdistended whatever method is selected. (In other words, manual expression requires constant vigilance; and tube drainage, whether by urethral or suprapubic catheter, must be continuous, never intermittent. Expression must be done at regular intervals; catheterization must be continuous. The retained catheter, furthermore, must never be shut off.)

THE LOWER TRACT

1. Make methylene blue and Gram stains on the discharge from every patient and repeat on three different occasions before deciding that the infection is not due to gonorrhea.

2. Make a darkfield examination at least twice on every penile lesion before applying any cauterizing substance which may mask or destroy the spirochetes temporarily.

3. Perform Wassermann test on the blood about six weeks after any penile lesion, no matter how soon this may have healed and regardless of the history.

1. Don't pass a catheter or other instrument into an infected urethra unless it is an emergency procedure to relieve retention or to examine an acute condition in the upper part of the tract.

2. Don't return a patient who has a urethral discharge to contact with others until the discharge has been proved by three examinations to be nonvenereal.

3. Don't allow patients to treat themselves with hand injections for any urethral infection unless it is impossible to provide for their treatment by qualified persons.

DO

4. Use the greatest gentleness and the greatest asepsis in passing a catheter or any instrument into the urethra.

5. Examine the scrotum and perineum carefully for evidence of extravasation in all cases of trauma and repeat this examination at frequent intervals.

6. Treat extravasation of urine into the scrotum or perineum by radical drainage with multiple incision and the urine diverted by cystostomy or external urethrostomy as indicated.

7. Perform exploratory operation in cases in which torsion of the testis is suspected.

DON'T

4. Don't discharge a patient suffering from stricture of the urethra. Have him return for periodic dilatations.

5. Don't do urethral irrigations, instrumentation, or rectal examination during acute epididymitis unless absolutely necessary.

6. Don't discharge any patient who has had gonorrhea until he has been thoroughly checked over and observed for a period of at least one month.

INDEX

ABDOMEN, great vessels, bleeding from, 15
injuries, upper, operation and, 44
inspection, in injuries, 23
"silent," 29
wall, in sealing of visceral wounds, 17
Abdominal approach to esophageal wound, 67
to kidney, 154
block, 182
hemorrhage, temperature in, 29
incisions, closure, 59
injuries, complications, 121–128
evisceration after, 98
patient status in, 21–36
operation in abdominothoracic injuries, 108
palpation in bladder rupture, 142
in kidney damage, 137
wall, foreign bodies, care, 59
in kidney damage, 151
injury, pain in, 21
vessels, perforation, 15
Abdominoscopy, 34
Abdominothoracic injuries, 107
wound, high, operation and, 44
Abrasions, bullet wounds and, 24
Abscess, hepatic, 93
in lesser peritoneal sac in stomach wounds, 72
in urethra injury, 205
intramural, 64
pancreatic, 98
perinephritic, care, 104
peritoneal, localized, drainage, 67
residual, 124
drainage, 58
examination for, 29
in abdominal injuries, 16, 122
subphrenic, x-ray in, 33
Acetic acid in tidal irrigation, 197
Acidophilus milk for soldiers, 19
Acidosis from mandelic acid, 147
Acriflavine in bladder rupture, 183
Adhesive tape suspensory for scrotum, 212

Aerograms in bladder rupture, 180
in bladder wounds, 175
Air hunger in abdominal injuries, 23
in peritoneoscopy, 34
raids, crushing injuries in, 163
Alcohol injection of lumbar sympathetic ganglia, 99
Alcoholism in bladder rupture, 175
Alimentary organs, hollow, wounds, 67
Alkalis in crush syndrome, 166
Alpha-lobeline, postoperative, 116
Aluminum alloys in armor, 18
Amino acids in nitrogen balance, 116
Ammonium chloride in urinary infection, 147
Amputation in crush syndrome, 165, 166
Anaerobic infection, postoperative, 117
Anastomosis, intestinal, mechanical, 77
of severed ureter, 167
of ureter, 104
of wounded esophagus, 69
Anemia in abdominal injuries, 122
in kidney injury, 137
Anesthesia, 47–50
effect on abdominal bleeding, 56
on liver bleeding, 92
on shock, 115
in bladder rupture, 181
protection against anaphylaxis, 41
Aneurysm in iliac vessel injury, 99
Angulation of intestine in repair, 76
Anorectal wounds, 29
Anoxemia in anesthesia, 49
Antiseptics for abdominal wounds, 62
in urethra injuries, 208
urinary, 201
Antitoxin therapy, preoperative, 40
Anuria in bladder rupture, 142
Anus, artificial, in cecum injuries, 79
avulsion, 85
Apathy in abdominal injuries, 23
Apparatus for continuous tidal irrigation, 198
Appearance, general, in abdominal injuries, 23
Appendicitis, sulfonamides in, 58

Apprehensive rigidity, 28
Armor in protection of abdomen, 18
Arterial disease in abdominal injuries, 122
Asbestos armor, 18
Ascending colon injuries, 80
Ascorbic acid, postoperative, 118
Asphyxia in crush injuries, 164
Aspiration, exploratory, of rectovesical abscess, 127
  in intraperitoneal bladder rupture, 185
  in tension pneumothorax, 109
  of subphrenic abscess, 125
Atelectasis in abdominal injuries, 121
  postoperative, 118
Atonic neurogenic bladder, 190
Atropine, preanesthetic, 47
Auscultation in abdominal injuries, 29
Automatic bladder, development, 195
Automobile accidents, bladder rupture in, 175
Autotransfusion in operations, 52
Avitaminoses in abdominal injuries, 122
  postoperative, 118
Avulsion of poles of kidneys, 101
  of spleen, 94
Azochloramid in abdominal wounds, 62

BACILLI in urinary infection, 146
Bacillus perfringens in wool clothes, 59
Back wounds, treatment, abdominal operation and, 55
Bacteria in urinary infection, 146
Bacteriologic studies in abdominal injuries, 32
Bacteriostatic substances for abdominal wounds, 62
  intraperitoneal instillation, 58
Bakelite armor, 18
Balata armor, 18
Ballottement in abdominal injuries, 29
Barbiturates, preanesthetic, 47
Base hospital, urography in, 138
Bile duct, injury, pancreas and, 96
  wounds, 87
  from torn liver, 93
Biliary peritonitis, 93
Bladder, automatic, 190
  capacity, cystitis and, 192
  catheterization, 169
  diseases, rupture and, 175
  distention in spinal cord injuries, 24
  tenderness in, 28

Bladder, emptying in warfare, 19
  injuries, 26, 72, 84, 104
    do's, don't's, 221
    war, 173–186
  mechanism, nerves in, 188
  neurogenic, care, 187–202
    do's, don't's, 222
  rupture, 141
    urethra and, 144
  tenesmus in abdominal injuries, 23
  wounds, extraperitoneal, 143
Blast injury, effect on abdomen, 24
  of liver, 90
  wave colonic injuries, 79
  concussion of small intestine, 74
Bleeding, external, in abdominal injuries, 24
  in kidney injury, control, 156
  in rectal injury, 84
  intraperitoneal, subperitoneal, externally, 15
  points, location, 55
  postoperative, in stomach wounds, 72
Block, abdominal, 182
Blood clots in sealing of visceral wounds, 17
  renal, x-ray and, 140
  counts in abdominal injuries, 31
  diastase in pancreas injury, 96
  extravasation in urethra injury, 206
  intraperitoneal, cleansing, 57
  lipase in pancreas injury, 96
  loss, operative, 115
  plasma in shock, 37
  pressure, effect of transfusion, 38
    in abdominal injuries, 30
    in crush syndrome, 164
    in visceral injury, 17
    spinal anesthesia and, 48
  specific gravity in abdominal injuries, 31
  studies in abdominal injuries, 30
    in bladder rupture, 143
    in crush syndrome, 164
    in kidney injury, 137
  sugar in pancreas injury, 96
  sulfonamides, peritoneal instillation and, 58
  supply of intestine, repair and, 76
  transfusion, 37
    continuous, 38
    during operation, 51, 52
    postoperative, 115
  urea in crush syndrome, 165

Blood vessels, great, abdominal, bleeding from, 15
  injuries, 27
  injury, pancreas and, 96
  major, injuries, 99
  mesenteric, injury, 88
  omental, injury, 90
  pelvic, injury, 26
  renal, wounds, 101
Blowing wounds, 107
Blunt force liver wounds, 90
  pressure injury of pancreas, 96
Body heat, preservation, in shock, 37
  injuries, abdominal injuries and, 121
Bone injury to colon, 78
  necrosis in bladder wound, 106
  spicule in rectum, 84
Boric acid in continuous tidal irrigation, 197
Bovine serum albumin, 116
Bowel emptying in warfare, 19
  in sealing of visceral wounds, 17
Bracing of patient in operation, 51
Bradycardia in abdominal injuries, 27
Brain, injuries, neurogenic bladder in, 188
Breathing exercises, postoperative, 118
Bronchoscopy, postoperative, 118
Bruises of colon, 78
Bulb catheter in suprapubic cystostomy, 201
Bullet injuries of small intestine, 72
  wounds from, 24
Burns in abdominal injuries, 121
Buttocks, injury, intraperitoneal wound and, 25
  wound, 85
    bladder and, 174

CAFFEINE sodiobenzoate in shock, 40
  sodium benzoate, postoperative, 116
Calculi in bladder wound, 106
  in cystitis, 192
  in pelvis fracture, 146
Calculus in ureter wound, 104
Calices, deformity, on x-ray, 140
  gunshot wounds, 150
Canvas, compressed, armor, 18
  in closure of abdominal wounds, 61, 62
Catgut in abdominal wounds, effect, 59
  in kidney hemorrhage, 104
Catheter, gastro-intestinal, 78
  indwelling, in urethra injury, 203
  retention, 196
    care, 199

Catheter, urethral, in bladder rupture, 183
Catheterization in bladder rupture, 142, 180
  wound, 175
  in kidney conditions, 217
    injury, 151
  in urethral rupture, 145
    wound, 144
  in urinary retention, 190
  intermittent, 187
  ureteral, in kidney injury, 153
Cecostomy, value, 84
Cecum injuries, 79
  perforation, pain and, 21
Celioscopy, 34
Celiotomy, 43
  after effects, 115
  exploratory, 85
    mortality in, 130
Cellophane for abdominal wounds, 60
Cerebral edema, oxygen in, 116
Chain mail armor, 18
Chemotherapy in catheterization, 142
  in incrusted cystitis, 140
  in neurogenic bladder, 201
  in urinary infection, 146
Chilling in operation, 51
  operative, 115
Cholecystectomy, 87
Cholecystoduodenostomy, 87
Cholecystogastrostomy, 87
Cholecystojejunostomy, 87
  in pancreas injury, 96
Cholecystostomy, 87
Chordee, breaking, 205
Chromium steel in armor, 18
Clamps in colostomy, 83
  on renal vessels, 103
Cleancut liver wound, 90
Closure, delayed, 60, 62
  incomplete, 62
  of abdominal incisions, 59
  through-and-through, 62
Cloth, cotton, in closure of abdominal wounds, 62
Clothing, intraperitoneal, 57
Coagulation in visceral injury, 17
Cocci in urinary infection, 146
Collapse, pain and, 22
Collateral circulation of mesentery, 88
Colon, exposure, 54
  herniation, 99
  injuries, 57, 69, 72, 78
    kidney and, 101
  repair, 76

Colon, pelvic, injury, 26
    perforation, infection and, 16
    spleen and, 94
    suturing to parietal peritoneum, 82
    wounds, liver and, 90
Color of bowel, resection and, 77
    of torn liver, 91
Colostomy, 82
    in rectal wound, 85
    mortality in, 84
    proximal, complete, 82
Composure in abdominal injuries, 23
Compresses in urethral injuries, 208
Compression atrophy of testicle, 212
    injuries of abdomen, pain in, 22
    of abdominal vessels, 56
Concussion, neurogenic bladder in, 188
Concussive renal injury, 136
Connell suturing of intestine, 75
Conservative treatment in kidney
    wounds, 103
Constriction of penis, 204
Contamination in abdominal injuries,
    121
    in evisceration, 98
Contusions of bladder, 173
    of kidney, 150
    of penis, 203
    of small intestine, 74
    of urethra, 205
Coramine in shock, 40
    postoperative, 116
"Cord" bladder, 188
Cork armor, 18
Corpuscular volume, in abdominal in-
    juries, 31
Costal arch, excision, 53, 54
    omental extrusion, 98
Cotton armor, 18
    sutures, 61
Course of projectiles, 24
Crateriform wounds of liver, 90
Crepitation, palpation for, 28
Crush syndrome, 163, 170
    kidney in, 102
Crushing bladder rupture, 175
    injury, renal failure and, 163
    of bowel, resection in, 77
Cul-de-sac abscess, 127
Curvilinear incision, 54
Cushing suturing of intestine, 75
Cushioning of patient in operation, 51
Cyanosis in abdominal injuries, 23
    in muerte subperiotoneal, 27
Cyclopropane anesthesia, 49
    barbiturates and, 47

Cystitis in bladder wound, 106
    incrusted, 148
    pyelonephritis and, 192
Cystography, excretory, in bladder
    wounds, 175
    injection, in bladder rupture, 180
    injection, in bladder wounds, 175
    retrograde, 33
        in bladder rupture, 143
Cystoscopy, bladder rupture in, 143,
    176
    in abdominal injuries, 33
    in atonic bladder, 193
    in bladder rupture, 180
    wound, 175
    in incrusted cystitis, 148
    in kidney injuries, 136, 137
    in kidney injury, 153
    in spastic bladder, 193
Cystostomy, suprapubic, 106, 183, 184
    in penile injury, 203
Cystotomy in bladder injuries, 221

DEATH, hypotension and, 38
    rate in hemorrhage, 15
        in viscera perforation, 15
    subperitoneal, 27
Débridement of wounds, 58
    in rectal wounds, 85
Decapsulation of kidneys in crush syn-
    drome, 166
Decubital ulcers in neurogenic blad-
    der, 187
    in spinal injuries, 192
Defecation in abdominal injuries, 23
Defects in parietes, palpation for, 28
Defunctionalization of bowel, 83
Dehydration in abdominal injuries, 122
    postoperative, 116
Demineralization in abdominal in-
    juries, 122
    postoperative, 116
Descending colon injuries, 80
Desert warfare, armor and, 18
Desoxycorticosterone acetate in shock,
    40
Detachment of mesentery, 88
    of omentum, 90
    of spleen, 94
Detrusor muscle, bladder, 189
Devine colostomy, 83, 84
Devitalization of intestine, 88
Diaphragm injuries, 107, 111
    kidney and, 155
    mobility, x-rays and, 32
    wound, operation and, 54

Diaphragmatic hernia in abdominal injuries, 122
Digital compression of abdominal vessels, 56
examination of rectum, 84
Disruption of kidney, 101
of spleen, 94
Distention, abdominal, in wounds, 24
bladder, injury and, 173
rupture and, 175
in liver hemorrhage, 92
of bladder, 142
of intestine, injury and, 74
overflow and, 187
vesical, 191
Diuresis, alkaline, in crush syndrome, 165
Diverticulectomy, bladder wall repair in, 176–177
Divisions of colon, 78, 80
of small intestine, 73, 74
of splenic pedicle, 94
Do's and don't's, 217–223
"Double barrel" resection, 77
Drain in ureter wound, 104
Drainage in bladder injuries, 106, 175
in colon wounds, 82, 84
in kidney injuries, 103
in pancreas injury, 96
in urethral injuries, 208
in urinary extravasation, 154
of bile, 93
of iliac fossa abscess, 127
of kidney, 170
of localized peritoneal abscess, 67
of peritoneal cavity, 58
of renal region, 155
of residual abscesses, 124
of scrotum in extravasation of urine, 206
of urinary accumulation, 167
extravasation, 168
of wounds, 64
suprapubic, 185
Dressings of chest wall, 109
Dribbling, 188
Drowsiness in abdominal injuries, 23
Drug therapy for shock and hemorrhage, 40
Drugs, stimulant, during operation, 52
postoperative, 116
Dulness, shifting, in abdominal injuries, 29
Duodenum, bile duct injury and, 86
injuries, 57, 72
gallbladder and, 87

Duodenum, injuries, pancreas and, 96
perforation, infection and, 16
wound, mortality, 78
Duration of crush syndrome, 165
of foreign bodies in abdomen, 57
of kidney drainage, 156
of operation, 64
of shock, 15
of urinary retention, 190
Dyspnea in abdomino-thoracic injuries, 23, 107
Dysuria, 192
in urethra injury, 205

ECCHYMOSIS in urethra injury, 206
of scrotum, 212
Edema in evisceration, 98
in visceral injuries, 44
intestinal mucosa, value, 17
limb, in crushing, 163
proteins and, 116
Elective dependence in visceral injury, 17
nonoperative management, 44
Electrovibrators for foreign bodies, 33
Embolism, postoperative, 118
Emphysema of penis, 203
subcutaneous, in abdominal injury, 28
Emptying of bladder, nerves and, 189
Empyema in abdominal injuries, 122
Encystment of foreign bodies, 67
End to end anastomosis, 77
Endoaneurysmorrhaphy, 100
Endoscopic examination in abdominal injuries, 33
Enema in bladder rupture, 181
in rectal atony, 201
postoperative, 117
Ephedrine in shock, 40
postoperative, 116
Epididymitis, traumatic, 213
Epididymo-orchitis, 213
Epidural anesthesia, 48
Epigastric arteries, deep, perforation, 15
Epinephrine in abdominal block, 182
in shock, 40
postoperative, 116
Epiploic appendix in colon wound repair, 82
foramen, digital compression near, 56
Épluchage of wounds, 58
Erosions in abdominal injuries, 122

Erythrocyte volume, 31
Eserine in ileus, 117
Esophagoscopy in abdominal injuries, 33
Esophagus, division, repair, 68
  exposure, 54
  injury, vomiting in, 22
  wounds, 67
Ether in abdominal injuries, 49
  irrigation of wounds, 63
Ethylene gas anesthesia, 49
Evacuation hospital, urography in, 138
  of urine and blood, 104
Eventration, 98
Eversion, intestinal mucosa, value, 17
Evisceration following abdominal injury, 98
  in small intestinal injury, 75
  pain in, 22
Excitement in abdominal injuries, 23
  pain and, 21
Excretory urogram, 138
Exploration in bladder rupture, 142
  in kidney injury, 154
  in penetration, 35
  in peritoneal wounds, 67
  in small intestinal wound, 75
  of thorax, 110
Explosive wound of bladder, 105
Exposure in abdominal injuries, 121
  in shock, 14
  mortality and, 130
  operative, 115
Exteriorization of small intestine, 77
External evidence of genito-urinary injuries, 138
Extirpation of adrenals, 98
Extraperitoneal bladder rupture, 141
  wound, 173
  wounds, treatment, 106
  colonic injury, 80
  lumbar nephrectomy, 159–162
  mass in bladder rupture, 142
  rectal wound, 85
  rupture of bladder, 177
  wounds of bladder and urethra, 143
Extravasation of intestinal contents, 74
  of urine, 142
  in bladder rupture, 179
Exudate in visceral injuries, 44
  peritoneal, sulfonamide absorption and, 58

FALLING drop apparatus, 39
Fatigue in shock, 15

Fecal fistulas, 84
  spontaneous, recovery in, 17
Feces, discharge, in abdominal injuries, 24
  from urethral wound, 144
  intraperitoneal, 57
Fever in kidney injury, 137
  in liver hemorrhage, 92
  in urethra wound, 206
Fiber armor, 18
Fibrin in sealing of visceral wounds, 17
Filling of bladder, nerves and, 188
Fish liver oil gauze packing, 62
  ointment in abdominal wounds, 62
Fissures of liver, 90
Fistulas, colonic, 79
  in abdominal injuries, 122
  intestinal drains and, 58
  vitamins and, 118
  pancreatic, 97
  ureteral, 104
  urinary, 205
  treatment, 167
Flank, blood in, in spleen injury, 94
  dulness, 29
  prominence, in abdominal injuries, 24
Flax armor, 18
Flora, intestinal, in protection of wounds, 18
Fluids in bladder rupture, 181
  in crush syndrome, 166
  in urinary infection, 147
  injection in bladder rupture, 143
  peritoneal, examination, 29
Flushes, postoperative, 117
Flushing of abdominal cavity, 186
Foley urethral catheter, use, 197
Food in stomach wounds, 72
  viscera perforation and, 16
Foreign bodies in kidney injuries, 155
  intraperitoneal, 57
  kidney, x-ray and, 141
  palpation for, 28
Foroblique cystoscope, 34
Fowler's position, postoperative, 115
Fracture, bladder rupture and, 177
  of pelvis, 145
  of penis, 203, 204
  wound of liver, 91
Fragmentation of liver, 90
Fragments in abdominal wound, 24
  in small intestinal injuries, 74
  stomach wounds from, 69
Friability of liver, 90

Fulguration of bladder, rupture in, 176
Furrowing of kidney, 149
Furrows of kidney, 101
    of liver, 90

GALLBLADDER wounds, 87
Gangrene in urethra wound, 206
Gas bacillus infection in abdominal in-
        juries, 28, 121
    distention in kidney injury, 152
    escape in stomach wound, 70
    gangrene in buttocks wound, 85
    in retrograde cystography, 143
    injuries in abdominal injuries, 121
    subdiaphragmatic, pain in, 22
    subphrenic, x-rays and, 32
    through abdominal wound, 32
Gastric juice, pain from, 21
Gastroduodenal catheter in ileus, 117
Gastroenterostomy in stomach wounds,
    71
Gastrohepatic omentum, compression,
    93
Gastroscopy in abdominal injuries, 33
Gastrostomy in esophageal division, 69
Gauze packs in hepatic bleeding, 57
    of liver, 92, 93
Genito-urinary injuries, 134–223
    organs, wounds, 100
        distal to bladder, 106
    tract injuries, survey, 135–148
        lower, injuries, do's, don't's, 222
Glucose in shock, 38
    postoperative, 116
Gluteal tear in rectal wound, 85
Glycogenesis, cortical extract and, 117
Gonorrhea, do's, don't's, 223
Gramicidin in peritonitis, 58
Gum armor, 18
Gunshot wounds of kidney, 149
    of ureter, 166

HAIR armor, 18
Handling of small intestine, 75
Harpooning method of localization, 33
Head-down position in shock, 37, 51
Head injuries, 121
Healing of ureter injuries, 171
Heat in bladder rupture, 181
    in contusion of penis, 203
    in urethra injuries, 208
    tent, postoperatively, 115
Helium, postoperative, 116
Hematemesis in stomach injury, 22
    in stomach wound, 70
Hematocele, operation in, 213

Hematocrit in abdominal injuries, 31
Hematoma, abdominal, crepitation in,
    29
    in abdominal injuries, 24
    in bile duct wounds, 87
    in colon wounds, drainage, 82
    in kidney injury, 102
    in urethra rupture, 144
    inguinal, 105
    mesenteric, in intestinal injury, 76
        in small intestinal wounds, 73
    obscuring, abdominal, 56
    of mesentery, central, 88
        peripheral, 87, 89
    of omentum, 90
    of penis and scrotum, 204
    perirenal, 102, 170
        evacuation, 155
    retroperitoneal, 16
        pancreas wound and, 96
    scrotal, 145
    subcapsular kidney, 101
        splenic, 94
    subcutaneous, of penis, 203
Hematuria in bladder wound, 105
    in kidney damage, 151
        injury, 136
            treatment, 154
    in renal injury, 102
    in ureter injury, 167
    in urethral wound, 144
    in urinary retention, 191
Hemisection of kidneys, 101
    of spleen, 94
Hemoconcentration, 30, 31
    in crush syndrome, 164
Hemoglobin studies in abdominal in-
        juries, 31
Hemoperitoneum, peritoneoscopy and,
    34
Hemorrhage, abdominal, pain and, 21
    anesthesia and, 47
    arrest, 55
    blood pressure and, 30
    death rate and, 15
    during operation, 51
    in abdominal injuries, 21, 121
    in bladder rupture, 179
        wound, 105, 174
    in blood vessel injuries, 99
    in colon wounds, 80
    in kidney injury, 102
        secondary, 151
    in liver injury, 91
    in mesentery tear, 88
    in partial nephrectomy, 156

Hemorrhage in penis wound, 156
  in peritoneal wounds, 67
  in small intestine, 74
  in splenic rupture, 94
  in stomach wounds, 70
  in visceral injury, 17
  intraperitoneal, pain in, 22
  postoperative, 115
  secondary, from liver, 91
    in kidney injury, 102
  shock and, 14
  treatment, 37
  visceral, spontaneous arrest, 17
Hemostasis, spontaneous, in liver, 92
Hemothorax in abdominothoracic in-
    juries, 107
Hemp armor, 18
Heparinization in splenectomy, 96
  postoperative, 118
Hepatic artery, compression, 93
  digital compression, 56, 57
  bleeding, 56
  flexure, repair, 80
  ligament in esophageal wound, 67
Hernia, diaphragmatic, 111
  x-rays and, 32
Hilum, kidney, wounds, 150
"Hockey-stick" incision, 109
Hospitalization of abdominal injuries,
    130
Hunger in shock, 14
Hydrogen   peroxide   in   abdominal
    wounds, 63
Hydronephrosis in neurogenic bladder,
    192
Hypertension in crush syndrome, 165
Hypogastric nerve to bladder, 188
Hypogastrium wound, bladder and, 174
Hypoproteinemia   in   abdominal   in-
    juries, 122
  postoperative, 115

IDENTIFICATION of bacteria in urinary
    infection, 146
Ileotransverse colostomy in intestinal
    injury, 77
Ileum injuries, 72
  perforation, infection and, 16
  wound, mortality, 78
Ileus, adynamic, in abdominal injuries,
    121
  adynamic, in evisceration, 22
  from glucose, 117
  in abdominal wounds, 24
  plasma in, 115
  postoperative, 77, 117

Iliac arteries, injuries, 99
  fossa abscess, 127
  mass, 29
Immobilization   in   epididymo-orchitis,
    214
  of wounds, 64
Implantation of ureter in bladder, 104
Incidence of abdominal injuries, 129
  of abdominothoracic injuries, 107
  of bladder wounds, 104
  of colon wounds, 78
  of gunshot wounds of kidney, 149
  of wounds of kidney, 100
    of liver, 90
    of pancreas, 96
    of rectum, 84
    of spleen, 94
    of small intestine, 72
    of stomach, 69
Incision, abdominal, types, 52
  for cecum injury, 81
  for renal exploration, 157
  in bladder operations, 184
  in extravasation of urine, 207
Incisions in abdominothoracic injuries,
    109
  in bladder operations, 184
    wounds, 106
  in colon injuries, 81
  in exploration of renal fossa, 155
  in kidney injury, 103, 154, 170
  in liver wounds, 93
  in lower ureteral injury, 169
  in penile hematoma, suppuration,
    203
  in peritoneoscopy, 34
  in spleen injury, 94
  in stomach wounds, 71
  in subphrenic abscess, 124
  in suprapubic cystostomy, 183
Incontinence, 188
  overflow, 190
  passive, 191
Indigocarmine in ureteral damage, 167
Infarction in small intestinal injuries,
    73
  of large intestine, 78
  of renal vessels, 101
Infection in abdominal injuries, 16
  in bladder wounds, 175
  in kidney injury, 152
  in neurogenic bladder, 195
  in urinary tract, 146
  in urogenital injuries, 107
  manual expression of urine and, 196
  renal, prevention, 194

Infection, urinary, in neurogenic bladder, 192
Inferior vena cava, injury, 99
Infusion during operation, 52
Infusions in shock, 38
    postoperative, 116
Inhalation anesthesia, 49
Injection of lumbar sympathetic ganglia, 100
Injuries, abdominothoracic, 107
    associated, in abdominal wounds, 21
    diaphragmatic, 111
    genito-urinary, 134–223
    intraabdominal, location, repair, 57
    of bladder, 173–186
    of gallbladder, 87
    of kidney and ureter, 149–171
    of kidneys, do's, don't's, 218
    of mesentery, 87
    of penis, urethra, scrotum, prostate, seminal vesicles, 203–215
    of prostate gland, 214
    of scrotum, 211
    of seminal vesicles, 214
    of testicle, 211
    of urethra, 205
    of vas deferens, 214
    shock in, 14
    to great omentum, 90
    to kidney, 135
    to major blood vessels, 99
Inspection of small intestine injuries, 75
Instrumentation, bladder rupture in, 176
    injury of urethra, 205
Insulin in glucose infusions, 39, 117
Intermittent irrigations of bladder, 199
Interrupted sutures, 61
Intestinal distention, bladder rupture and, 141
    fistulas, bladder and, 142
    ileus in hemorrhage, 16
    obstruction, drains and, 58
        postoperative, 117
    resection in mesenteric injury, 90
Intestine, contents, spilling, 16
    injury, bladder and, 104
    kidney gunshot wounds and, 149
    large, wounds, 78
    small, extrusion, 99
        injuries, kidney and, 101
        wounds, 57, 69, 72
            colon and, 79
    tear from mesentery, 88
    wall, bleeding, 16

Intestine, wounds, closing, 75
Intra-abdominal operations, genito-urinary injuries and, 135
Intraperitoneal bladder rupture, 141
    wound, 173
    colonic injury, 80
    hemorrhage, 16
    perforation of bladder, 105
    rectal wound, 85
    rupture of bladder, 176
Intravenous anesthesia, 49
Intubation, intestinal, 78
Inverted-V incision for bladder, 183–185
Iodides in retrograde cystography, 143
Irrigation of wounds, 63
Irritability of bladder, 147
Ischemia from mesenteric hematoma, 87, 88
    in crush injuries, 164
    of lower extremities, 100

JAUNDICE in liver injury, 91
Jejunostomy in esophageal division, 69
    in stomach wounds, 72
Jejunum injuries, 72
    perforation, infection and, 16
    wound, mortality, 78

KAPOK armor, 18
Kidney, colon injury and, incision in, 81
    exposure, 54
    failure in crushing injury, 163
    fossa, exploration, 155
    function, nephrectomy and, 153
    gunshot wounds, 149
    healing, x-ray and, 140
    hemorrhage, 15
    in crush syndrome, 165
    injuries, 135, 149–166
        adrenal and, 98
        vomiting in, 22
    nontraumatic injuries, do's, don't's, 217
    parenchyma, wounds, 149
    pedicle, rupture, 137
    repair, 156
    sepsis in neurogenic bladder, 187
    wounds, liver and, 90
        spleen and, 94

LABORATORY studies in abdominal injuries, 21, 30
Lacerated wound of small intestine, 73

Lacerations of kidney, 101, 150
  of penis, 203
  of rectum, 84
  of small intestine, 74
  of urethra, 205
Lactobacilli in soldiers, 19
Laminated metal in armor, 18
Laparoscopy, 34
Laparotomy, exploratory, 35
Laryngospasm, cyclopropane and bar-
  biturates causing, 47
Lavage of peritoneal cavity, 58
  of wound of abdominal wall, 59
Layered closure, 60
Leakage, external, of urine, 102
Leather armor, 18
Legs in pelvis fracture, 146
Lembert suturing of intestine, 75
Lesions of colon, 79
Ligaments in operation on kidney,
  160
Ligation of bleeding points, cotton in,
  61
  of iliac arteries, 99
  of iliac vessel, 100
  of mesentery, 89
  of omentum, 90
  of ureteral stump, 167
Ligatures, nonabsorbable, 59
Linear stomach wound, 69
Liver abscess, x-ray in, 123
  approach, 110
  dulness in abdominal injuries, 29
  exposure, 54
  functions, vitamins and, 118
  hemorrhage, 15, 44
  herniation, 99
  injuries, 57, 69, 72, 90
  injury, operation and, 44
  kidney gunshot wounds and, 149
  necrosis, sulfonamides and, 58
  wounds, kidney and, 101
Local anesthesia in abdominal injuries,
  49
Loin incisions, 54
  wound, colon and, 81
  wounds, hematuria in, 151
Lower extremity wounds, urethra and,
  143
Lumbar approach to kidney, 154
  plexus, trauma, pain in, 22
  sympathetic ganglia, injection, in
    iliac artery injury, 99
Lumen of bowel, resection and, 77
Luminal occlusion, proteins and, 116
Luxation of testicle, 213

MACHINISTS' cotton waste pressure
  dressing, 63
Mandelic acid in neurogenic bladder,
  201
  in urinary infection, 147
  in urogenital injuries, 107
Manganese steel in armor, 18
Manual expression of urine, 187, 195
Marsupialization of traumatic pseudocyst, 97
Mass in bladder rupture, 179
  reflex in manual expression of urine,
    196
Meatus bleeding in urethra rupture,
  144
  urethral, inspection, 145
Mediastinitis in esophageal injury, 69
Melena in abdominal injuries, 23
Mesenteric artery, superior, digital
  compression, 55
  blood vessels, bleeding from, 15
  vessels, crushing, 79
Mesentery, injuries, 57, 87
  in small intestinal injuries, 73
  tears, approximation, 75
  effect on colon, 79
Metrazol in shock, 40
  postoperative, 116
Micturition, automatic, 190
  in bladder wound, 105
  nervous centers and, 189
  periodic reflex, 191
Midline incision, 53
Milk, intraperitoneal infection and, 16
Miller-Abbott tube, postoperative, 117
Missiles, intraabdominal, x-rays and,
  32
  lodgment, pain and, 22
Mobile unit for shock and hemorrhage,
  39
Mobilization of colon, 81, 82
  of splenic flexure, 80
  of ureter, 104
Morphine, abdominal pain and, 22
  effect on rigidity, 28
  in shock, 37
  postoperative, 115
  preanesthetic, 47
Mortality, anesthesia and, 48
  degree of hemorrhage and, 14
  duration of operation and, 64
  in abdominal injuries, 17, 129-131
    wounds, factors affecting, 18
  in abdominothoracic injuries, 112
  in bladder rupture, 180
    wounds, 106

Mortality, celiotomy, 130
 colon wounds, 84
 in gastric wounds, 72
 in hepatic wounds, 94
 in intestinal resection, 76
 in kidney wounds, 104
 in pancreas injury, 98
 in rectal wounds, 85
 in small intestinal wounds, 78
 in splenectomy, 96
 in splenic injury, 96
 nonoperative, 29
 time of operation and, 43
Motility of bowel, resection and, 77
Motorized equipment, armor and, 18
Movement of abdomen in injury, 23
Mucosa in gastric wounds, 70
 in small intestinal wounds, 73
 intestinal, eversion, edema, effects, 17
Muerte subperitoneal, 27
Multiple diameters method of localization, 33
Murphy button, obstruction and, 77
Muscle destruction, renal failure in, 163
 gap, palpation for, 28
 hypertrophy in neurogenic bladder, 193
 in operation on kidney, 158
 necrosis in crush syndrome, 164
 pad in liver repair, 92, 93

NATURAL protective mechanisms, 17
Nausea in abdominal injuries, 22
 in kidney injury, 102
"Nearest point" localization, 32
Neck pain in abdominal injuries, 22
Necropsy in warfare, 129
Neglect of neurogenic bladder, 187
Nembutal, preanesthetic, 47
Nephrectomy, 103, 156
 in renal artery injury, 150
 in urinary fistula, 167
 lumbar, extraperitoneal, 159–162
 partial, 156
 technic, 158
 transabdominal, 155
Nephrostomy, 167
 in ureter wound, 104
Nerves, abdominal incisions and, 53
 in bladder mechanism, 188
 in limb crushing, 163
 in operation on kidney, 159
 injury, neurogenic bladder in, 188
Net wire, armor, 18

Neurogenic bladder, care, 187–202
 do's, don't's, 222
Nicotinic acid amides, postoperative, 118
 postoperative, 118
Nitrogen equilibrium, 116
Nitrous oxide anesthesia, 49
Noncatheterization in neurogenic bladder, 187, 195
Nonoperative management, in visceral injury, 17
Note of exclamation wound of stomach, 69
Number of small intestinal wounds, 72

OBLIQUE incisions, 53, 54
Obstruction, mechanical, neurogenic bladder and, 193
 to ureteral catheterization, 167
Occlusion of vas deferens, 214
Oliguria in kidney injury, 137
Omentum approach in stomach wounds, 71
 extrusion, 98
 grafting in colon wounds, 82
 great, injuries, 90
 in bladder rupture, 142
 in sealing of viscereal wounds, 17
 injury, bleeding from, 15
Openings in stomach wounds, 69
Operation, blood pressure and, 30
 exploratory, in bladder rupture, 180
 for rupture of urethra, 209, 210
 in bladder rupture, 181
 in stomach wound, 71
 selection of patients for, 43–45
Operative procedure, in abdominal injuries, 51–65
 order of, 55
Oral hygiene, intraperitoneal infection and, 16
Orchidectomy, 213
Organs, effect on shock, 15
 herniated through diaphragm, 111
 injury, bladder injury and, 174
 shock and, 15
 solid, hemorrhage from, 15
 wounds, 67–113
Orthodiagraphic method of localization, 33
Overdistention of neurogenic bladder, 187
Oxygen during operation, 52
 in anesthesia, 49
 postoperative, 116
 therapy in shock, 40
"Oyster complex," armor and, 18

PACKING in kidney bleeding, 156
in liver wounds, 93
of splenic wound, 96
with bacteriostatic solution, 62
Pain, colicky, in kidney injury, 102
in abdominal wounds, 21
in abdominothoracic injuries, 107
in bladder rupture, 141, 178
in bladder wound, 174
in kidney injury, 136
in liver hemorrhage, 92
in manual expression of urine, 196
in stomach wounds, 70
relief, in shock, 37
Pallor in abdominal injuries, 23
in liver hemorrhage, 92
Pancreas injuries, gallbladder and, 87
pseudocysts in abdominal injuries, 122
wounds, 96
Paper armor, 18
Parallax method of localization, 32
Paralytic bladder, care, 187
Paramedian incision, 53
Parasympathetic nerve to bladder, 189
Parenteral fluids, blood studies and, 30
effect on blood, 31
Parker-Kerr end-to-end anastomosis, 77
Patient, attention, during operation, 51
care, in abdominal injuries, 37–41
in hopeless condition, 43
not requiring operation, 44
position in kidney operation, 157
selection for operation, 43–45
status in abdominal injuries, 21–36
Pelvic cellulitis in bladder wound, 106
colon injury, 78, 80, 84
floor injuries, abdominal rigidity in, 28
nerve to bladder, 189
Pelviostomy, 167
Pelvis, abscesses in, 29
fracture, bladder rupture in, 142, 175
wound in, 173
colon wounds and, 80
urethra injury in, 205
rupture and, 145
injury, bladder and, 104
kidney, injury, 150
renal, tear, x-ray in, 140
Penetration, exploration in, 35
hollow viscera, sealing, 17
in abdominal wounds, 21
of kidney, 135

Penicillin in peritonitis, 58
Penis in urethral rupture, 144
injuries, 203
semierection, in muerte subperitoneal, 27
Penrose drains in kidney region drainage, 155
Pentamethylenetetrazol in shock, 40
Pentobarbital in bladder rupture, 181
Pentothal sodium in induction of anesthesia, 47
intravenously, 49
Percussion in abdominal injuries, 29
Perforation in gastric wounds, 72
of bladder, 105
of colon, 78, 80
of kidney, 101, 150
of liver, 90
of mesentery, 87
of rectum, 84
of small intestine, 72
repair, 76
of spleen, 94
of viscera, death rate and, 15
Peridural anesthesia, 48
Perineal slough, 206
Perinephritic accumulations, 103
Perineum, extravasation of urine, 179
in urethral rupture, 144
infection in rectal wound, 85
injury, intraperitoneal wound and, 25
pain in urethral rupture, 144
wound, bladder and, 174
Perirectal extraperitoneal space infection, 85
Perirenal density in x-ray, 138
hematomas, 103
hemorrhage, 136
mass, palpation of, 137
urine, 140
Peritoneal cavity, cleansing, 57
cavity, drainage, 58
lavage, 58
wounds, 67
contamination in abdominal injuries, 21
irritation in liver injury, 91
in spleen injury, 94
in stomach wounds, 70
tears of kidney, 150
urine, 167
Peritoneoscopy, 34
Peritoneum injury, pain in, 22
perforation, 35
shock and, 15

Peritoneum, suture in kidney injury, 103
wounds, 67
Peritonism, traumatic, 137
Peritonitis, autolytic, 93
chemical, 93
in abdominal injuries, 24, 67, 121
in bladder rupture, 142, 179
wounds, 106
in rectal wound, 85
postoperative, 117
Perivesical hematoma, 106
Perspiration in abdominal injuries, 23
Pfannenstiel curved incision for bladder, 184
Phenobarbital in bladder rupture, 181
Phlebothrombosis, 115
in abdominal injuries, 122
Phosphoric acid in tidal irrigation, 197
Phrenic nerve in diaphragm surgery, 112
left, crushing, in esophageal anastomosis, 69
Physical examination in abdominal injuries, 23
Pituitary extract in adynamic ileus, 117
in shock, 37, 40
postoperative, 116
Placing of patient in opedation, 51
Plane, right angled, method, of localization, 33
Planographic method of localization, 33
Plasma, postoperative, 115
proteins, 31
specific gravity, 31
Plastic armor, 18
operations on kidney, 156
repair of kidney, 170
Pleura injury in nephrectomy, 162
Pleural cavity injury, kidney gunshot wounds and, 149
Pneumonitis, postoperative, 118
Pneumothorax in abdominothoracic injuries, 107
Polyvalent serum in abdominal injuries, 41
Portal vein, compression, 93
digital compression, 56, 57
Position in abdominothoracic trauma, 108
Positive pressure anesthesia, 49
Posterolateral incision for kidney, 158
Postoperative care of gastric injuries, 72

Postoperative treatment, 115–119
Post-traumatic kidney secretion, 152
Posture, effect on course of projectiles, 24
Potassium citrate in crush syndrome, 166
permanganate in intermittent irrigations, 199
in urethra injuries, 208
Preanesthetic preparation, 47–50
Preoperative preparation, 37–41
in bladder rupture, 181
Presacral areolar tissue injury, 85
Pressure dressings of wounds, 64
wave, clothing and, 18
Priapism in spinal cord injury, 201
Procaine in abdominal block, 182
injection of lumbar sympathetic ganglion, 99
Proctoscopy in abdominal injuries, 33
Projectiles, course, 24
intraperitoneal, 57
pain from, 22
Prostate gland, bladder rupture and, 175
injury, 27, 206, 214
bladder and, 104
Prostigmine methyl sulfate in ileus, 117
Protective mechanisms, natural, 17
Pseudocyst, excision, 97
in pancreas injury, 96
Pseudohydronephrosis on x-ray, 140
Psoas margin in perirenal bleeding, 152
muscle, outline, in kidney damage, 102
Psychoses in abdominal injuries, 121
Pudic nerve to bladder, 189
Pulmonary edema, oxygen in, 116
lesions, postoperative, 118
Pulse in abdominal injuries, 27
in muerte subperitoneal, 27
spinal anesthesia, and, 48
Punctate injuries of liver, 90
of spleen, treatment, 96
Puncture of omentum, 90
of urethra, 205
wound of penis, 204
of small intestine, 73
Purse-string ligature of rectum, 85
suturing of intestine, 75, 76
Pyelography in kidney damage, 103
retrograde, 137
in kidney injury, 153
Pyelonephritis in neurogenic bladder, 192

Pyelo-ureterography, intravenous, 33
Pyridine betacarboxylic acid diethyl-
    amide in shock, 40

RAGGED wounds of liver, 90
Rayon armor, 18
Recovery, natural protective mechan-
    isms and, 17
    spontaneous, in visceral injury, 17
Rectal examination in abdominal in-
    juries, 29
    in bladder rupture, 143
    in urethral rupture, 145
    tenesmus in abdominal injuries, 23
Rectovesical abscess, 124, 127
    pouch, suturing, 85
Rectum activity, neurogenic bladder
    and, 201
    injuries, 26, 72, 84
        bladder and, 104
        colostomy in, 82
Reflection of colon, 81
Reflex bladder, 191
Regeneration of scrotum, 211
Regional block anesthesia, 49
Reimplantation of ureter, 167
Relaxing sutures in esophageal anas-
    tomosis, 69
Renal artery injury, 150
    colic, injury and, 136
    function, injury and, 137
    pelvis, injuries, 101
        visualization, 138
    torsion, x-ray in, 139
Repair in bladder wounds, 175
    of mesenteric injury, 89
    of urethral wounds, 208
Resection in small intestinal wounds,
    73, 76
    of colon, 82, 84
    of omentum, 90
    of pancreas, 97
    of small intestine, multiple, 76
    omental, in evisceration, 99
Residual urine, 193
Respiration, effect on liver bleeding,
    92
    on visceral injuries, 25
    rapid, in abdominal injuries, 23
    spinal anesthesia and, 48
Rest in contusion of penis, 203
    in kidney injury, 152
    in shock, 37
    in urethra injuries, 208
Restlessness in abdominal injuries, 23
Retention, 188

Retention, catheter, 187
    urinary, 190
Retrograde pyelogram, 138
Retroperitoneal hematomas, 121
    perforation of colon, 78
Rib fracture, diaphragm injury in, 111
    liver wounds in, 90
    spleen wound in, 94
Riboflavin, postoperative, 118
Ribs in operation on kidney, 160
Rigidity, alternating, in abdominal in-
    juries, 28
    in abdominal injuries, 28
    in abdominothoracic injuries, 107
    in bladder rupture, 141
    in renal damage, 151
    in stomach wounds, 70
    in superficial wounds, 25
    lumbar muscles, in kidney injury,
        102
Ringer's solution, lactated, in shock,
    38
    postoperative, 116
Roentgenoscopic control, intermittent,
    for foreign bodies, 33
Roentgenoscopy in abdominal injuries,
    32
Rubber in armor, 18
    tissue drains, 60, 64
Ruddock peritoneoscope, 34
Rupture of bladder, 141, 173, 175
    spontaneous, 175
    of colon coats, 78
    of kidney, 136
    of urethra, 144, 205, 208
    traumatic, kidney, 150

SACRAL region, injury, intraperitoneal
    wound and, 25
Sacrum wound, 85
Saline, azochloramid in, 62
    hypertonic, in shock, 40
    in peritoneal lavage, 58
    in shock, 38
    irrigation of wounds, 63
    postoperative, 116
Scopolamine, preanesthetic, 47
Scores of kidney, 101
Scrotum, hematoma, 204
    in urethral rupture, 144
    injuries, 211
    slough, 206
Sea sponge pressure dressing, 64
Seconal, preanesthetic, 47
Sedation, preanesthetic, 47
Semiflexion in operation, 51

Seminal vesicles, injury, 214
Sepsis in abdominal injuries, 122
  in bladder rupture, 179, 181
    wounds, 106
  in colon wounds, 84
  in kidney injury, 103
  in loin wounds, 82
  of retroperitoneal tissues, 87
Serum albumin in shock, 37
  polyvalent, postoperative, 117
  protein in abdominal injuries, 31
Severance of penis, 203
  of ureter, 167
Sexual function in neurogenic bladder, 202
Shattering of kidney, 150
  of liver, 90
Sheet metal armor, 18
Shell caps, pain from, 22
  fragments, pain from, 22
Shock, anesthesia and, 47
  "cart," portable, 39
  conditions affecting, 14
  during operation, 51
  effect on blood, 31
  hemorrhage and, 14
  in abdominal injuries, 21, 121
  in abdominothoracic injuries, 107
  in bladder rupture, 142, 178
    wound, 174
  in crush syndrome, 164
  in evisceration, 98
  in intestinal repair, 76
  in kidney injury, 102, 151
    treatment, 153
  in peritoneal bleeding, 30
    lavage, 58
  in spleen injury, 94
  in urethra rupture, 144
  kidney secretion in, 152
  operation and, 44
  operative, 115
  postoperative, 115
  primary, 38
  secondary, 38
  spinal anesthesia and, 48
  treatment, 37
Short circuiting in intestinal injury, 77
Shrapnel injuries of kidney, 150
Side to side anastomoses, 77
Sigmoid mesentery hematoma, 89
Sigmoidoscopy in abdominal injuries, 33
Silicon nickel steel in armor, 18
Silk sutures, 61
Silver nitrate in incrusted cystitis, 148

Silver nitrate, administration in injuries to urethra, 208
Sinus tachycardia in abdominal injuries, 40
Sinuses, from nonabsorbable sutures, 59
  in abdominal injuries, 122
Sisal armor, 18
Site of intraperitoneal bladder rupture, 177
Skin flaps in abdominal wounds, 62
  markers, localization and, 32
  palpation, in abdominal injuries, 27
  undermining, by bullets, 24
Sleep, loss, in shock, 14
Slits in small intestinal wounds, 74
Small intestine, separation from mesentery, 74
  wounds, 84
Sodium bicarbonate in crush syndrome, 166
  citrate in tidal irrigation, 197
  sulfate in crush syndrome, 166
  tetradecyl sulfate in azochloramid, 62
Solid viscera, wounds, 90
Somatic nerve to bladder, 189
Spastic neurogenic bladder, 190
Specific gravity of blood, 31
Spermatic cord, injury, 106, 211
Sphincter division in rectal wound, 85
  muscle, bladder, 189
Spillage in colon wounds, 84
  rigidity in, 28
  visceral, pain and, 21
Spilling in small intestinal wounds, 74
  in visceral injury, 16
Spinal anesthesia, 47
    continuous, 48
    in bladder rupture, 181
  column injury, spinal anesthesia and, 48
  cord, abdominal injuries and, 24
    injury, neurogenic bladder in, 188
      paralytic bladder in, 187
Spine deviation in perirenal bleeding, 152
  kidney gunshot wounds and, 149
Spleen, exposure, 54
  hemorrhage, 15, 44
  injuries, 57, 69, 72, 94
  wounds, kidney and, 101
Splenectomy, 95
Splenic flexure, repair, 80
Splits in splenic capsule, 94
  of colon, 80

Splits of liver, 90
Stainless-steel wire sutures, 61
Starvation, mortality and, 130
Statistics, mortality, 129–131
Status of bladder, neurogenic, 195
    of patients in abdominal injuries,
    21–36
Stellate liver wounds, 90
Stereoscopic x-rays, 32
Stimulants in bladder rupture, 181
Stoma, enteric, formation, 77
Stomach, esophageal anastomosis to,
    69
    herniation, 99
    injuries, 57, 69, 72
        vomiting in, 22
    perforation, spilling in, 16
    prolapse, 69
    wall, bleeding, 16
    wounds, colon and, 79
        liver and, 90
        spleen and, 94
"Stove in" chest wall, 107
Straddle injuries of urethra, 145
Strain in shock, 14
Strangulation in evisceration, 98
    of extruded bowel, 99
Strength loss in liver hemorrhage, 92
Streptococci in urinary infection, 146
Strictures in urethral injuries, 208
    of ureter, 104
    specific, wounds, 67–113
Subcostal incisions, 53
    in colonic flexure injury, 81
    in esophageal wound, 67
    in spleen injury, 94
Subdiaphragmatic abscess in stomach
    wounds, 72
Subhepatic abscess in stomach wounds,
    72
Subparietal renal injury, 135
Subphrenic abscess, 29
    anterior, 126
    posterior, 124
    x-ray in, 123
Sucking wounds, 107
Suction drainage in gastric injuries,
    72
    in abdominal hemorrhage, 56
    in ileus, 117
    of bladder clots, 136
    of mucus in air passages, 118
    tube in extraperitoneal rupture, 186
Sulfanilamide in abdominal injuries, 37
    in urinary infection, 147
Sulfapyridine in urinary infection, 147

Sulfathiazole in urinary infection, 147
Sulfonamides in abdominal injuries, 37
    in contaminated wounds, 62
    in neurogenic bladder, 201
    in postoperative pneumonitis, 118
    in prevention of peritonitis, 19
    in urogenital injuries, 107
    intraperitoneally, 58
    postoperative, 117
    toxicity, 122
Suppuration of penis, 203
Suprapubic cystostomy, 183, 187
        continuous tube drainage and, 200
    drainage, 185
    exploration in bladder rupture, 143
    suction apparatus, 199
Suprarenal cortical extract, postopera-
    tive, 117
    cortical hormone in shock, 40
    glands, wounds, 98
Surgery, bladder rupture in, 176
    in kidney injury, 219
    in rupture and wounds of bladder,
    185
    procedures for wounds of kidney, 155
Survival rate in abdominothoracic in-
    juries, 112
Susceptibility to shock, 15
Sutures in intestinal resection, 77
    nonabsorbable, 59
    of "blowing" thoracic wound, 109
    of gallbladder, 87
    of kidney, 103
    of spleen, 95
Suturing in bladder wounds, 106
    in drainage of kidney, 156
    in kidney bleeding, 156
    in liver wounds, 93
    of colonic wounds, 82
    of diaphragm, 112
    of inferior vena cava, 99
    of mesentery, 89
    of ureters, 104
Swelling in liver hemorrhage, 92
Sympathetic nerves to bladder, 188
Sympathetic-parasympathetic balance
    in bladder, 189
Symptoms in abdominothoracic in-
    juries, 107
    of injuries of large intestine, 80
    of small intestinal injuries, 75

TABES dorsalis, cord bladder in, 188
Tabetic bladder, rupture, 178
Tears of colon, 78, 80
    of kidney capsule, 101

Tears of kidney, x-ray in, 153
  of mesentery, 87
  of omentum, 90
  of spleen, 94
  of ureter, 167
Telephone probes for foreign bodies,
  33
Temperature in abdominal injuries,
  27, 29
  of infusions, 116
Tenderness in abdominal injuries, 27
  in abdominothoracic injuries, 107
  in bladder rupture, 141, 179
  in kidney injury, 102, 136, 151
  in rectal wound, 85
  in stomach wounds, 70
Tenesmus in abdominal injuries, 23
Tension pneumothorax, 107
Testicles, injury, 211
  luxation, 213
  pain, in abdominal wound, 22
Tetanus antitoxin in abdominal injuries, 40
  toxoid in abdominal injuries, 40
Thigh, extravasation of urine, 179
  injuries, abdominal rigidity in, 28
  intraperitoneal wound and, 25
Thirst, in shock, 14
Thoracic injuries, head-down position
  in, 51
  wall wound, operation and, 54
  wounds, anesthesia and, 49
  esophagus in, 67
Thorax injuries, abdominal rigidity in,
  28
Thrombin in hepatic hemorrhage, 57
  topical, in liver bleeding, 93
Thrombophlebitis, 115
  in abdominal injuries, 122
  postoperative, 118
Thrombosis of mesenteric vessels in
  small intestinal injuries, 73, 77
  postoperative, 118
  progressive, in splenectomy, 96
Through-and-through injury of thorax,
  108
Tidal irrigation, continuous, 196
Time for nephrectomy, 157
  in abdominal injuries, 21, 44
  interval in manual expression of
  urine, 195
Tissues, effect of urine, 157
  urine extravasation in, 168
Tomographic method of localization,
  33
Tonus in automatic micturition, 191

Tourniquets in shock, 37
Transabdominal approach to kidney,
  155
Transperitoneal nephrectomy, 170
Transpleural approach to abdomen,
  109
  to liver, 93
Transpleural-transdiaphragmatic exposure, 110, 111
Transportation delay, mortality and,
  130
Transversalis fascia in kidney operation, 158
Transverse colon injuries, 79
  incisions, 53, 54
Trauma, operative, 115
Trendelenburg position in bladder rupture, 183
  in pelvic colon injuries, 82
Triacetin, azochloramid in, 62
Triangular ligament, in urethra rupture, 144
Triangulation methods of localization,
  33
Tubes, irrigating, in abdominal closure,
  60
  suprapubic, 201
Tumors, desmoid-like, of abdominal
  wall, 62

ULCERATION in gastric wounds, 72
  of colon mucosa, 79
Umbilical tape in esophageal wound,
  67
Umbilicus, bluish, in peritoneal hemorrhage, 24
Uremia in crush syndrome, 164
  in urethra rupture, 208
Ureter displacement in kidney damage,
  103
  gunshot wounds, 166
  in kidney injury, x-ray and, 153
  injuries, 26, 204, 150, 166–171
  do's, don't's, 220
  severance, 102
Ureteral catheters in kidney damage
  218
Ureteropyelograms, excretory, 152
Ureterostomy, 167
Urethra, injuries, 205
  posterior, injury, 26, 106
  rupture, 144
  straddle injuries, 145
  stricture, bladder rupture in, 175
  wounds, extraperitoneal, 143
Urethral catheter, use, 135

Urethral instrumentation, bladder
    wound in, 173
Urethrogram, 145
Urethrostomy, perineal, 106
Urgency, 192
    of kidney treatment, 153
Urinal in manual expression, 196
Urinary antiseptics, 107
    extravasation, 144
    infection in abdominal injuries, 122
    leakage in ureteral wound, 166
    tract, infection, 146
Urine cultures, 147
    discharge, in abdominal injuries, 24
        in bladder wound, 105
    examination, 169
    extravasation, 152
        in bladder wound, 174
    in abdominal injuries, 30
    in crush syndrome, 164
    in kidney injury, 102, 137
    manual expression, 195
    reaction in chemotherapy, 147
    retention in kidney injury, 136
        in urethral injury, 206
        in urethral rupture, 144
Urogram, excretory, in kidney injury,
    152
Urography, 137
    in bladder rupture, 143
    intravenous, in bladder rupture, 180
Uterus, injuries, 100

VALVULAR colon wounds, 80
    stomach wound, 70
Vas deferens, injury, 211, 214
Vasa deferentia, injury, 106
Vascular suture, 99
Vaseline gauze for abdominal wounds,
    60
Venereal diseases, do's, don't's, 223
Ventroscopy, 34
Vermin, armor and, 18
Vertical incisions, abdominal, 53
Vesical irrigations in rupture, 181
    neck resection, bladder rupture in,
        176
        rupture, 186
Vinethene anesthesia, 49
Violence, indirect, to small intestine,
    74
Viscera, damage, in kidney injury, 154
    detached parts, intraperitoneal, 57
    in abdominal wound, 24
    injury, effect of position, 25
        in abdominothoracic wounds, 107

Viscera, injury, pulse in, 27
    spontaneous recovery in, 17
    perforation, death rate and, 15
    infection and, 16
    peritoneoscopy and, 34
    solid, wounds, 90
Vitamin B$_1$, postoperative, 118
Voiding, desire, in bladder rupture,
    141, 179
Vomiting in abdominal injuries, 22
    in abdominothoracic injuries, 107
    in kidney injury, 102
    in stomach wound, 70
V-type stomach wound, 70

WAR injuries of bladder, 173–186
    of genito-urinary tract, 135–148
Wassermann test in penile lesion, 223
Water blast wave abdominal injuries,
    22, 23
"Water-hose kink" intestinal obstruc-
    tion, 117
Wheals in crush syndrome, 164
Wire mesh armor, 18
Wounds, beveling of edge, 58
    débridement, 58
    drainage, 64
    épluchage, 58
    healing, blood proteins and, 116
        vitamins in, 118
    immobilization, 64
    infections in abdominal injuries, 122
        postoperative, 117
    irrigation, 63
    of bladder, 104, 173
    of entrance, 24
        in bladder injury, 104
        peritoneoscopy and, 34
    of esophagus, 67
    of exit, 24
    of genito-urinary organs, 100, 106
    of hollow alimentary organs, 67
    of intestine, large, 78
    of kidneys, 100
        liver and diaphragm, 155
    of pancreas, 96
    of penis, 203
    of peritoneum, 67
    of rectum, 84
    of small intestine, 72
    of solid viscera, 90
    of specific structures and organs,
        67–113
    of spleen, 94
    of stomach, 69
    of suprarenal glands, 98

Wounds of testicle, 211
  of ureters, 104
  of urethra, 205
  omentum in, 24
  projectile course and, 24
  remote, in abdominal injuries, 23
  superficial, abdominal, 25
Woven silk armor, 18

X-RAY examination in abdominal injuries, 32

X-ray in abdominal injuries, 21
  in bladder injuries, 221
  in kidney conditions, 217
  in kidney injury, 102, 152, 169
  in subphrenic abscess, 123
  in ureteral injury, 220

ZINC peroxide paste for abdominal wounds, 60
  in anaerobic infection, 117
  in delayed closure, 63